Academy

C000180165

Eating Disorders
Second Edition

Jessica Setnick, MS, RD, CEDRD

Academy of Nutrition and Dietetics
Chicago, IL

eat right. Academy of Nutrition and Dietetics

Academy of Nutrition and Dietetics Pocket Guide to Eating Disorders, Second Edition

ISBN 978-0-88091-980-7 (print)
ISBN 978-0-88091-981-4 (ebook)

Catalog Number 436X17 (print)
Catalog Number 436X17e (eBook)

10   9   8   7   6   5   4   3

For more information on the Academy of Nutrition and Dietetics, visit www.eatright.org.

Contents

Reviewers

Ruth Leyse-Wallace, PhD, RDN
Alpine, CA

April Winslow, MS, RDN, CEDRD
San Jose, CA

Chapter 1
Eating Disorders and the Dietitian

Introduction

Whether it is in your patient population, among coworkers or colleagues, in family members or friends, or even in strangers, registered dietitian nutritionists (RDNs) are often the first to identify dysfunctional eating behavior. Whether or not the treatment of eating disorders falls within your specialty practice area, at some point in your career, you are bound to encounter situations that require your understanding of this complex issue. They are simply too common to avoid.[1]

Rough estimates suggest at least 13.5 million Americans meet criteria for anorexia, bulimia, or binge eating disorder.[1-4] A 2005 survey of 1,500 American adults reported that 4 of 10 either had or knew someone who had an eating disorder.[2] As an RDN, eating disorders may be more common among your peers than in the general community.[5,6] You may even have been motivated to enter the field because of past experiences with your own or a loved one's eating disorder.[7]

Sadly, only a small fraction of those with eating disorders ever enter, much less complete, treatment.[8] The reasons are many and include:

- denial of the illness and its severity (called anosognosia);
- fear that recovery will require weight gain or other undesirable consequences;
- feeling ashamed of behaviors and hiding them from fear of embarrassment;
- cost of treatment and inadequate insurance coverage; and

- general lack of awareness of eating disorders among those in the medical profession.

Because modern society's fixation on image and appearance can seem to condone, encourage, and reward pathological attempts at weight control, eating disorders are sometimes unnoticed until they are life threatening. A woman with anorexia is 12 times more likely to die at a young age[9] and 59 times more likely to commit suicide[10] than a woman of the same age without anorexia. Even in death, an eating disorder can remain undiagnosed, as the cause of death may be listed as a more immediate complication, such as heart failure or cardiac arrest.

Eating disorders do not discriminate. They afflict individuals of every race, age, and socioeconomic status. Although most research subjects to date have been female, the eating-disorder research community is slowly becoming more inclusive. Patterns may appear, but there is no "typical" eating disorder patient. It is dangerous and unethical for an RDN to rule out an eating disorder solely on the basis of gender, economic status, weight, age, appearance, mental capacity, or any other single factor.

Because nutritional rehabilitation is a cornerstone of eating disorder recovery,[11] your influence as an RDN is powerful.[1,12,13] Through education, you can raise awareness of the factors known to cause eating disorders and of their early warning symptoms; through assessment, you can identify eating disorders at their earliest stages; and through intervention, you can change the course of lives.

This book is intended to prepare you for when you encounter an individual with an eating disorder in your professional life. The Nutrition Care Process (NCP) format is followed throughout. The NCP is comprised of 4 steps and is outlined in detail in Appendix A; refer to Box 1.1 for a brief outline of the steps of the NCP.

Box 1.1 Nutrition Care Process[14]

Step 1—Nutrition Assessment
Nutrition assessment data have been organized into 4 domains:

- Food/Nutrition-Related History
- Anthropometric Measurements
- Biochemical Data, Medical Tests, and Procedures
- Nutrition-Focused Physical Findings
- Patient/Client History

Step 2—Nutrition Diagnosis
Nutrition diagnoses have been organized into 3 domains:

- Intake
- Clinical
- Behavioral-Environmental

Step 3—Nutrition Intervention
Nutrition intervention strategies have been organized into 4 domains:

- Food and/or Nutrient Delivery
- Nutrition Education
- Nutrition Counseling
- Coordination of Nutrition Care

Step 4—Nutrition Monitoring and Evaluation
Nutrition monitoring and evaluation outcomes are organized into 4 domains:

- Food/Nutrition-Related History Outcomes
- Anthropometric Measurement Outcomes
- Biochemical Data, Medical Tests, and Procedure Outcomes
- Nutrition-Focused Physical Finding Outcomes

Terminology

"Eating disorders" is the umbrella term currently used to describe abnormal and maladaptive eating and related behaviors with psychological and biological underpinnings. In the United States, the American Psychiatric Association (APA) oversees the establishment of criteria for defining psychiatric conditions. These are updated and published periodically in the *Diagnostic and Statistical Manual of Mental Disorders*, which is currently in its fifth edition (*DSM-5*).[15] Because the underlying cause or causes of eating disorders have not been confirmed, the current categorization of eating disorders is based on signs, symptoms, and behaviors. This system can be problematic, as individuals with similar or even identical symptoms may have different causative factors, different neurochemical imbalances, different disease processes, and different needs for treatment. This is one of the reasons why individualization of treatment is so essential.

In the *DSM-5*, more eating disorder types are described than ever before. These include anorexia nervosa, bulimia nervosa, binge eating disorder, avoidant/restrictive food intake disorder (ARFID), night eating syndrome, purging disorder, and others. Each have their own diagnostic criteria, some more detailed than others (see Boxes 1.2 through 1.6, pages 6–10).[15]

Five of these diagnoses are grouped into a category called "other specified feeding and eating disorders" (OSFED). These are purging disorder, night eating syndrome, "atypical" anorexia, and bulimia and binge eating disorder "of low frequency or limited duration." In the past, these might have been categorized as "eating disorders not otherwise specified" (EDNOS). As with EDNOS, it is important to note that OSFED is not an eating disorder in itself, and also that those eating disorders within the OSFED category should not be considered less severe eating disorders.

They simply are variations of eating disorders that are not as well-defined as some of the others. Further research is needed on all of the disorders in this category.

The *DSM-5* introduced another new category, "unspecified feeding and eating disorders." This is not an actual disorder but rather a diagnostic code that can be used when a practitioner is unable to determine the details of a patient's eating disorder, for example, if the individual is unresponsive, uncooperative, or mentally altered. It is intended simply to be a placeholder until more information can be gathered.

Etiology of Eating Disorders

Binge eating, self-induced vomiting, excessive exercise, starvation, and other eating disorder behaviors are harmful and destructive, so why do they begin, and why do they persist? The answers are under investigation, and there are no definite answers yet. The effects of eating disorders on the body and brain are far better understood than their causes. It appears that both genetic and environmental influences contribute to the development of eating disorders,[11] but because research is generally initiated after the onset of the eating disorder and sample sizes are often small, it is unclear how much each factor plays a role.

Biological Factors

Early family studies suggested some heritability of eating disorders,[16,17] and later studies showed genetic markers are similar among family members with anorexia.[18] Twin studies have suggested that genetic contributions toward eating disorders may change during puberty,[19] that boys with a female twin are more likely to develop an eating disorder than those with a male twin,[20] and that binge eating disorder and bulimia may share genetic factors.[21] Neonatal complications and the mother's health during pregnancy may also influence later eating disorder development.[22]

Box 1.2 *DSM-5* Criteria for Anorexia Nervosa

A. Restriction of energy intake relative to requirements, leading to a significantly low body weight in the context of age, sex, developmental trajectory, and physical health. Significantly low weight is defined as a weight that is less than minimally normal or, for children and adolescents, less than that minimally expected.

B. Intense fear of gaining weight or of becoming fat, or persistent behavior that interferes with weight gain, even though at a significantly low weight.

C. Disturbances in the way in which one's body weight or shape is experienced, undue influence of body weight or shape on self-evaluation, or persistent lack of recognition of the seriousness of the current low body weight.

Specify Type

Restricting

During the last 3 months, the individual has not engaged in recurrent episodes of binge eating or purging behavior (self-induced vomiting or the misuse of laxatives, diuretics, or enemas). This subtype describes presentations in which weight loss is accomplished primarily through dieting, fasting, and/or excessive exercise.

Binge eating/purging

During the last 3 months, the individual has engaged in recurrent episodes of binge eating or purging behavior (self-induced vomiting or the misuse of laxatives, diuretics, or enemas).

Specify Severity Based on Body Mass Index (BMI)

Mild: ≥ 17

Moderate: 16–16.99

Severe: 15–15.99

Extreme: < 15

Box 1.3 *DSM-5* Criteria for Bulimia Nervosa

A. Recurrent episodes of binge eating. An episode of binge eating is characterized by both of the following:

   (1) Eating, in a discrete period of time (eg, within any 2-hour period), an amount of food that is definitely larger than what most individuals would eat in a similar period of time and under similar circumstances.

   (2) A sense of lack of control over eating during the episode (eg, a feeling that one cannot stop eating or control what or how much one is eating).

B. Recurrent inappropriate compensatory behaviors in order to prevent weight gain, such as self-induced vomiting; misuse of laxatives, diuretics, or other medications; fasting; or excessive exercise.

C. The binge eating and inappropriate compensatory behavior both occur, on average, at least once a week for 3 months.

D. Self-evaluation is unduly influenced by body shape and weight.

E. The disturbance does not occur exclusively during episodes of anorexia nervosa.

Specify Severity Based on Average Number of Compensatory Behavior Episodes per Week

Mild: 1–3

Moderate: 4–7

Severe: 8–13

Extreme: 14 or more

Box 1.4 *DSM-5* Criteria for Binge Eating Disorder

A. Recurrent episodes of binge eating, characterized by both of the following:

(1) Eating, in a discrete period of time (eg, within any 2-hour period), an amount of food that is definitely larger than most people would eat during a similar period of time and under similar circumstances.

(2) A sense of lack of control over eating during the episode (eg, a feeling that one cannot stop eating or control what or how much one is eating).

B. The binge eating episodes are associated with three (or more) of the following:

(1) Eating much more rapidly than normal.

(2) Eating until uncomfortably full.

(3) Eating large amounts of food when not feeling physically hungry.

(4) Eating alone because of feeling embarrassed by how much one is eating.

(5) Feeling disgusted with oneself, depressed, or very guilty afterward.

C. Marked distress regarding binge eating is present.

D The binge eating occurs, on average, at least once a week for 3 months.

E. The binge eating is not associated with the recurrent use of inappropriate compensatory behavior and does not occur exclusively during the course of bulimia or anorexia nervosa.

Specify Severity Based on Average Number of Binge Eating Episodes per Week

Mild: 1–3

Moderate: 4–7

Severe: 8–13

Extreme: 14 or more

Box 1.5 *DSM-5* Criteria for Avoidant/Restrictive Food Intake Disorder

A. An eating or feeding disturbance (eg, apparent lack of interest in eating or food; avoidance of eating based on the sensory characteristics of food; concern about adverse consequences of eating) as manifested by persistent failure to meet appropriate nutritional and/or energy needs associated with one (or more) of the following:

   (1) Significant weight loss (or failure to achieve expected weight gain or faltering growth in children).

   (2) Significant nutritional deficiency.

   (3) Dependence on enteral feeding or oral nutritional supplements.

   (4) Marked interference with psychological functioning.

B. The disturbance is not better explained by lack of available food or by an associated culturally sanctioned practice.

C. The eating disturbance does not occur exclusively during the course of anorexia nervosa or bulimia nervosa, and there is no evidence of a disturbance in the way in which one's body weight or shape is experienced.

D. The eating disturbance is not attributable to a concurrent medical condition or not better explained by another mental disorder. When the eating disturbance occurs in the context of another condition or disorder, the severity of the eating disturbance exceeds that routinely associated with the condition or disorder and warrants additional clinical attention.

Reprinted with permission of the American Psychiatric Association. *The Diagnostic and Statistical Manual of Mental Disorders.* 5th ed. Arlington, VA: American Psychiatric Association; 2013.

Box 1.6 *DSM-5* Criteria for Other Specified Feeding and Eating Disorders

Atypical Anorexia Nervosa

All of the criteria for anorexia nervosa are met except that despite significant weight loss the individual's weight is within or above the normal range.

Bulimia Nervosa of Low Frequency and/or Limited Duration

All of the criteria for bulimia nervosa are met except that the binge eating and inappropriate compensatory behaviors occur on average less than once a week and/or for less than 3 months.

Binge eating Disorder of Low Frequency and/or Limited Duration

All of the criteria for binge eating disorder are met except that the binge eating occurs on average less than once a week and/or for less than 3 months.

Purging Disorder

Recurrent purging behavior to influence weight or shape (eg, self-induced vomiting; misuse of laxatives, diuretics or other medications) in the absence of binge eating.

Night Eating Syndrome

Recurrent episodes of night eating as manifested by eating after awakening from sleep or by excessive food consumption after the evening meal. There is awareness and recall of the eating. The night eating is not better explained by external influences such as changes in the individual's sleep-wake cycle or by local social norms. The night eating causes significant distress and/or impairment in functioning. The disordered pattern of eating is not better explained by binge eating disorder or another mental disorder including substance abuse and is not attributable to another medical disorder or to an effect of medication.

Regarding the perpetuation of eating disorder behaviors once they have begun, we are starting to understand that the neurochemical changes associated with eating disorder behaviors are similar to those induced by drugs of abuse.[23,24] This may explain why individuals with eating disorders often struggle with other addictions.[25] Eating disorders also co-occur with anxiety, depression, obsessive-compulsive disorder (OCD), post-traumatic stress disorder (PTSD), attention-deficit disorder (ADD), and borderline personality disorder (BPD),[15] but whether the connections are cause and effect, genetic, environmental, or all of these, is yet unknown. Connections have also been suggested between eating disorders and hormonal imbalances, including polycystic ovary syndrome (PCOS), hypoglycemia, and menstrual irregularities not specifically related to nutrition.

Nonbiological Factors

In addition to a biological susceptibility, the formation of most eating disorders seems to require some environmental stimulus. Eating disorders are often reported to develop in proximity to a weight change, whether intentional or unintentional; to be injury-, illness-, or catastrophe-related; or to develop as an aftereffect of an emotional shock.

It is well understood that restriction of energy intake leads to biochemical and psychological changes that resemble eating disorders.[26] What is not understood is why some individuals who undertake low-calorie diets develop eating disorders while others do not. Often the social effects of weight changes are dramatically negative or positive, so regardless of an individual's original intention to lose or gain weight, criticism or praise for doing so can trigger an eating disorder if the biological susceptibility exists.

In some cases, weight changes that lead to eating disorders are preceded by one or more physically or emotionally disorienting events, referred to in the mental health field as "emotional trauma."[27,28] It is unknown if the biochemical effects of starvation are more strongly felt by those in emotional distress. In these cases, the desire for weight loss may be a misplaced attempt to modulate stressful feelings and has been described as an effort to regain a sense of control.[11] Because of their effects on neurochemistry, eating disordered behaviors do, in fact, cause a temporary feeling of well-being. They create a positive feedback loop to perpetuate the behavior, even beyond the point where they become harmful or life-threatening.

The Dietitian's Role

RDNs contribute to many aspects of eating disorder treatment at every level of care.[29-35] Box 1.7 lists some of the functions an RDN may play in the treatment of eating disorders.

Am I Ready?

Every RDN has something to offer to an individual struggling with an eating disorder. The primary requirement is an interest in the field and willingness to learn. However, care of individuals with eating disorders is a specialty area of practice, and to be most effective, requires additional training beyond what is provided in school and internship programs.[15, 32-34, 36]

Therefore, if you are just starting to practice in this field, it is essential that you reach out to your supervisor, your treatment team, or a more experienced RDN for guidance. Also, you will want to focus your continuing education efforts on eating disorders and mental health. If you find yourself either doubting your abilities or "taking your work home with you," know these are common reactions, not signs that you are inadequate. Remember that the eating disorders field is filled with controversies and unanswered questions and that the diseases themselves have no known cure. Reach out for support from other dietitians, mental

Box 1.7 Role of the RDN in the Treatment of Eating Disorders

Evaluate the patient's current eating patterns and share findings with other team members. Develop an individualized plan for improvement to replenish nutritional deficiencies and promote optimal nutrition and growth.

Help the patient determine how to implement needed nutritional recommendations.

Identify dysfunctional and detrimental thoughts and feelings around food, eating, and body size, as well as knowledge and skill deficits that prevent the patient from implementing recommendations.

Explain the role of proper nutrition and eating in physical and mental well-being and provide education to challenge inaccurate beliefs about food.

Refer information about underlying life stressors to a mental health professional.

Offer active learning activities when appropriate, such as cooking, eating, or grocery shopping, to help teach new behaviors and acceptance of food-related tasks and environments. Model appropriate eating in shared experiential interventions such as restaurant meals.

Communicate frequently with other members of the interdisciplinary treatment team, including family members and significant others.

Educate parents and caregivers regarding eating disorders and nutrition as they relate to the treatment plan and recovery needs.

Teach group nutrition classes to patients, their families and caregivers, and lead group nutrition discussions that address dysfunctional eating and promote improved nutrition.

health professionals at your facility, or a support or networking group for eating disorder professionals, and seek out ongoing mentoring or supervision with a more experienced RDN or mental health professional.

If you realize that you are not interested in the field, you do not feel sympathetic toward individuals with eating disorders, or you get easily frustrated with slow or little progress, you may choose not to seek out this patient population. When you encounter an individual with an eating disorder, as you occasionally will regardless of your specialty, speak with your supervisor for guidance, refer the individual to a different RDN, and ensure that you have moral support to help you cope with what can be a stressful situation.

Even with an affinity for eating disorder treatment, you will encounter individuals whose needs exceed what you can provide. When you are not sure what advice to give, simply respond without judgment that you will help the individual find an appropriate professional to help with his or her current situation. Then consult with your colleagues on available resources or other professionals located in your area.

Finally, if you realize that you are struggling with your own eating issues, or if you recognize that your work is triggering unhealthy thoughts or behaviors, know that this does not disqualify you from work as an RDN. You do need to seek help, and you may choose not to work with this patient population for a period of time. It is not necessary to be a "perfect" eater in order to help others. To be able to care for both your patients and yourself, awareness of your own thoughts, stressors, and behaviors is needed, as well as active engagement in your own recovery. This assures that when you are with patients, you are able to meet their needs without disregarding your own and that you can keep your own eating issues separate from the needs of your patients. A meeting with an experienced mental health professional or RDN is a starting place to assess your own relationship with food and determine how to proceed. Although it is not recommended that you discuss your eating disorder or your recovery with your patients, you can silently be a role model, showing that difficulties can be overcome.

References

1. Bruce B, Wilfley D. Binge eating among the overweight population: a serious and prevalent problem. *J Am Diet Assoc*. 1996;96:58-61.
2. National Eating Disorders Association. American public opinion on eating disorders. Updated February 2010. http://med.stanford.edu/scopeblog/Statistics%20%20Updated%20Feb%2010%2C%202008%20B.pdf Accessed August 10, 2010.
3. Marcus MD, Wing RR. Binge eating among the obese. *Ann Behav Med*. 1987;9:23.
4. Spitzer RL, Devlin M, Walsh BT, et al. Binge eating disorder: a multisite trial for the diagnostic criteria. *Int J Eat Disord*. 1993;11:191-203.
5. Kinzl JA, Traweger CM, Trefalt E, Mangweth B, Biebl W. Dietitians: are they a risk group for eating disorders? *Eur Eat Disord Rev*. 1999;7:62-67.
6. Worobey J, Schoenfeld D. Eating disordered behavior in dietetics students and students in other majors. *J Am Diet Assoc*. 1999;99:1100-1102.
7. Hughes R, Desbrow B. Aspiring dietitians study: a pre-enrollment study of students' motivations, awareness, and expectations relating to careers in nutrition and dietetics. *Nutr Diet*. 2005;62:106-109.
8. Striegel-Moore RH, Leslie D, Petrill SA, Garvin V, Rosenheck RA. One year use and cost of inpatient and outpatient services among female and male patients with an eating disorder: evidence from a national database of insurance claims. *Int J Eat Disord*. 2000;27(4):381-338.
9. Sullivan PF. Mortality in anorexia nervosa. *Am J Psychiatry*. 1995;152:1073-1074.
10. Keel PK, Dorer DJ, Eddy KT, Franko D, Charatan DL, Herzog DB. Predictors of mortality in eating disorders. *Arch Gen Psychiatry*. 2003;60:179-183.

11. Yager J, Devlin MJ, Halmi KA, et al. *Practice Guideline for the Treatment of Patients with Eating Disorders.* 3rd ed. Arlington, VA: American Psychiatric Association; 2006.

12. Bruce B, Agras WS. Binge eating in females: a population-based investigation. *Int J Eat Disord.* 1992;12:365-373.

13. American Dietetic Association. Position of the American Dietetic Association: nutrition intervention in the treatment of anorexia nervosa, bulimia nervosa, and other eating disorders. *J Am Diet Assoc.* 2006;106(12):2073-2082.

14. Academy of Nutrition and Dietetics. *eNCPT: Nutrition Care Process Terminology.* Chicago, IL: Academy of Nutrition and Dietetics; 2014. http://ncpt.webauthor.com/pubs/idnt-en/

15. American Psychiatric Association. *The Diagnostic and Statistical Manual of Mental Disorders.* 5th ed. Arlington, VA: American Psychiatric Association; 2013.

16. Lilenfeld LR, Kaye WH, Greeno CG, et al. A controlled family study of anorexia nervosa and bulimia nervosa. *Arch Gen Psychiatry.* 1998;55:603-610.

17. Strober M, Lampert C, Morrell W, Burroughs J, Jacob C. A controlled family study of anorexia nervosa: evidence of familial aggregation and lack of shared transmission with affective disorders. *Int J Eat Disord.* 1990;9(3):2339-2253.

18. Grice DA, Halmi KA, Fichter MM, et al. Evidence for a susceptibility gene for anorexia nervosa on chromosome 1. *Am J Hum Genet.* 2002;70(3):787-792.

19. Klump KL, Burt SA, McGue M, Iacono WG. Changes in genetic and environmental influences on disordered eating across adolescence: a longitudinal twin study. *Arch Gen Psychiatry.* 2007;64(12):1409-1415.

20. Procopio M, Marriott P. Intrauterine hormonal environment and risk of developing anorexia nervosa. *Arch Gen Psychiatry.* 2007;64(12):1402-1407.

21. Wade TD, Bulik CM, Sullivan PF, Neale MC, Kendler KS. The relation between risk factors for binge eating and bulimia nervosa: a population-based female twin study. *Health Psychol.* 2000;19(2):115-123.

22. Favaro A, Tenconi E, Santonastaso P. Perinatal factors and the risk of developing anorexia nervosa and bulimia nervosa. *Arch Gen Psychiatry.* 2006;63:82-88.

23. Wang G, Volkow ND, Thanos PK, Fowler JS. Similarity between obesity and drug addiction as assessed by neurofunctional imaging: a concept review. *J Addict Dis.* 2004;23(3):39-53.

24. Kalra SP, Kalra PS. Overlapping and interactive pathways regulation appetite and craving. *J Addict Dis.* 2004;23(3):5-21.

25. Helfman BL, Dennis AB. Understanding the complex relationship between eating disorders and substance use disorders. *Renfrew Perspect.* 2010;(Winter):2-4.

26. Kalm L, Semba R. They starved so that others be better fed: remembering Ancel Keys and the Minnesota experiment. *J Nutr* 2005;135(6):1347–52.

27. Berg FM. *Women Afraid to Eat: Breaking Free in Today's Weight-Obsessed World.* Hettinger, MD: Healthy Weight Network; 2000.

28. Vredrvelt P, Newman D, Beverly H, Minirth F. *The Thin Disguise: Understanding and Overcoming Anorexia and Bulimia.* Nashville, TN: Thomas Nelson; 1992.

29. International Association of Eating Disorder Professionals. *The CEDRD in Eating Disorder Care.* Pekin, IL: International Association of Eating Disorder Professionals; 2015.

30. Position of the American Dietetic Association: Nutrition intervention in the treatment of anorexia nervosa, bulimia nervosa, and other eating disorders;

31. American Dietetic Association. Nutrition intervention in the treatment of eating disorders. *J Am Diet Assoc.* 2006;106(12):2073-82.

32. Tholking MM, Mellowspring AC, Eberle SG, et al. American Dietetic Association standards of practice and standards of professional performance for registered dietitians (competent, proficient, expert) in disordered eating and eating disorders. *J Am Diet Assoc.* 2011;111:1242- 1249.e37

33. Reiter CS, Graves L. Nutrition therapy for eating disorders. *Nutr Clin Pract.* 2010;25:122-136.

34. Sloan R. The role of the registered dietitian in eating disorder treatment: a reality check. *SCAN's Pulse.* 2011;30(4):11-12.

35. Setnick J, Johnson M. Interventions used in nutrition counseling for eating disorder treatment: survey results. *SCAN's Pulse.* 2012;31(3):12-14.

36. Trammell EL, Reed D, Boylan M. Education and practice gaps of registered dietitian nutritionists working with clients with eating disorders. *Top Clin Nutr.* 2016;31(1).73-85.

Chapter 2

Nutrition Assessment for Eating Disorders

Inpatient Versus Outpatient Settings

Depending on the setting in which you work, as a registered dietitian nutritionist (RDN) you will encounter individuals with eating disorders in varying stages of illness, recovery, and motivation to change.

Inpatient and Residential Treatment

In a treatment center or hospital, your thorough nutrition assessment of an individual with an eating disorder will help determine the care plan and the goals set by the treatment team and should be performed as soon as is reasonable after admission. Medically unstable patients may require nutrition support on an emergency basis before a more thorough nutrition assessment can be performed, and patients who are extremely malnourished, uncooperative, or hostile (such as those who are hospitalized against their will) may need time to adjust before meeting productively with you. In these cases, draft a preliminary nutrition assessment using information available to you from medical records, family members, and other care providers until you can meet with the individual himself or herself.

Outpatient

In an outpatient setting, your nutrition assessment will initially rely on information provided by the patient, available family members or caregivers, and the referring

professional, if there is one. You may find differences of
opinion regarding severity, frequency, and duration of
symptoms. In these cases, the nutrition assessment may
actually take place over the course of several meetings.

Interviewing Patients

RDNs may encounter patients with eating disorders who
are comfortable with treatment and welcome your assistance. Other patients resent their need for an RDN's help or
carry a grudge from a past bad experience. The latter may
require more time to "warm up" to you and to participate in
your assessment. Patients who are ashamed of their eating
habits may not be forthcoming about specific behaviors or
may minimize or deny their eating disorder because of fear
of punishment or other negative consequences. They may
need a few sessions with you to build a relationship and rapport before determining that you are dependable and worth
trusting.

Asking about an individual's past experiences with treatment and treatment providers and allowing him or her to
express what he or she did and did not like about past providers can be informative. Resist the urge to mentally or
verbally agree with derogatory remarks made about past
caregivers or treatment programs. Keep in mind that effective eating disorder treatment can be difficult, painful, and
even involuntary; therefore a patient may harbor negative
memories of what was in fact excellent treatment. However, if you are concerned that an individual's report of past
treatment indicates a violation of law or ethical conduct,
speak with your supervisor, who can follow your facility's
procedures for this type of situation.

In some cases, your initial nutrition assessment will be
the first time an individual has ever spoken about his or her
eating disorder or spoken about it to a professional. These
situations carry additional significance, as the patient's

experience of this encounter has the potential to influence his or her willingness to pursue recovery in general. With this type of patient, your expressions of compassion and hope may be as important as the nutrition information you convey.[1,2] Your referrals to additional care are also of utmost importance (see Chapter 7). Do not collude with a patient in keeping the eating disorder secret if you believe that additional care is necessary. Seek advice from a supervisor or trusted colleague if an individual in this situation refuses additional care, especially medical attention.

You may observe that a patient responds differently to questions when accompanied by family members compared with when he or she is alone with you. You may find it beneficial to your understanding of the individual to discuss this observation with other treatment team members and to request their assistance determining a course of action.

Appropriate Terminology and Questions

During your initial assessment, use verbal and nonverbal cues from the patient to guide the length and depth of the meeting. Individuals who are very talkative may benefit from redirection ("That would be a great topic for your counseling session.") and guidance toward the information you need to gather ("I'm interested in hearing more about how that affects your eating."). Individuals who are very shy may be comforted by your assertion that eating is a personal topic and that you appreciate their willingness to speak with you.

Unless the patient is a medical professional, use general terminology during your assessment rather than technical or eating-disorder specific language (eg, "Do you ever feel guilty after you eat?" rather than "Do you purge?").[3] This will allow you to ask follow-up questions about the individual's specific behaviors (eg, "What do you do when you feel that way?" or "Do you do it every time that you eat or only in certain situations?") and also help avoid introducing new eating disorder behaviors to young patients. Every assessment should be tailored to the individual needs of the patient.

Suggested and sample questions are listed in Box 2.1. It is unlikely that you will need to ask all of these questions to any one individual. Some patients will give thorough answers; others will only answer the question directly asked. Pick and choose those questions that seem appropriate based on your preliminary knowledge of the patient's situation, and adapt as you continue. Some answers will require follow-up questions. Keep in mind that your goal is not to gather every possible data point on this individual but rather to obtain baseline information that you will use to make recommendations and build a rapport for future disclosure and trust as time goes on. If treatment goes as planned, you will meet with this patient many more times and continue to gather (and provide) information during each session.

Your interview will likely touch on all five categories in the Nutrition Assessment section of the Nutrition Care Process (see Box 1.1). The following sections explain how eating disorders interact with each Nutrition Assessment category.

Nutrition Assessment: Food/Nutrition-Related History

Assessment of Excess Intake

Alcohol (Includes Binge Drinking): Alcohol use is linked to disordered eating, even in the absence of alcohol dependence (alcoholism). Individuals who consume alcohol may skip meals or induce vomiting to compensate for percieved caloric intake.

Box 2.1 Sample Question Phrasing for Eating Disorder Assessment

"Can you bring me up to date on what brought you here?" If the patient denies having an eating disorder or states, "I'm only here because [someone else] thinks I have a problem," ask, "What is your understanding of why [that person] wanted you to be here?"

"Describe your eating on a typical day." Include timing and content of meals and snacks. If the patient specifies "on a good day…" or "on a bad day …" follow up on what, in the patient's opinion, makes eating "good" or "bad" and how often each type of day occurs. Include timing and quantities of noncaloric and nonnutritional food and beverage items, including abnormal intake of condiments, water, artificial sweeteners, coffee, chewing gum, alcohol, energy drinks, and so on.

"Are you allergic to any foods?…Are there other foods that you don't eat?…What are the reasons you don't eat those foods?"

"Do you ever worry that you'll get out of control around food and eat much more than you wanted to?…Is it just a worry, or does it sometimes happen?"

"Can you give me an example of what you might eat that feels like way too much?…How often does this happen?"

"What foods are your weakness?…Do you try to avoid them?… What happens when you are around them eventually?"

"Do you ever eat in secret?…How is it different than eating with others?"

"Do you wake up in the middle of the night to eat?…Are you awake when it happens or asleep?"

"Do you ever wake up to find evidence of eating that surprises you?"

"Do you ever have trouble keeping your food down?"

"Do you ever feel guilty after you eat?…How do you respond to that guilt?"

"Do you ever feel like you have to 'get rid of' your food?"

"Do you ever avoid eating when you are hungry?…Tell me more about that."

"Is there anything special you need to do with your food?…Any routines that you follow when preparing or plating your food or

Continued on next page.

Box 2.1 (cont.) Sample Question Phrasing for Eating Disorder Assessment

during a meal?" Examples include cutting food into many tiny pieces; reheating food during a meal; drawing out a meal for a certain length of time; eating only with certain dishware or flatware; measuring or weighing portions before eating; eating only a certain number of items at a time (eg, everything in threes); and other food "rituals." Ask about other eating disordered behaviors if not already described, such as sham eating, laxative use, compulsive weighing, and so on. Include frequency of behavior and any identifiable triggers ("Does it happen every time you eat, or only in certain situations?…What situations cause you to participate in that behavior?").

Ask about physical activity. If applicable, include frequency, duration, and type of exercise; compulsion to exercise ("Can you miss a day of exercise?"); secrecy of exercise ("Do you ever exercise even though you're not supposed to?"); relationship to eating ("Is your eating the same on a day you exercise and a day you don't exercise?"); exercise rituals ("Is there anything specific that you do every time when you exercise?"); as well as any recommendations from other health providers recommending or restricting physical activities.

Bioactive Substances: Drinking coffee (or ingesting instant coffee crystals or coffee beans), tea, caffeinated carbonated beverages, and energy drinks can result in an excessive intake of caffeine and other stimulants. Individuals may consciously use these stimulants to depress or mask appetite, maintain energy levels in the face of inadequate caloric intake, or propel excessive exercise. It is also possible that some individuals may be unaware of the role that such stimulants play in their eating disorder. Caffeine dependence may require a weaning process to prevent physical symptoms of withdrawal (the most notable is severe headache). Caffeine overuse may also indicate a form of self-medication for attention-deficit disorder (ADD) or chronic fatigue that merits medical evaluation. See Appendix C for caffeine content of common items (page 196).

Fortified Foods and Supplements Containing Vitamins and Minerals: Individuals attempting to reduce their intake of calories may choose processed foods over fresh or homemade foods simply because the processed foods seem more portion-controlled and the nutrition information more standardized. They may state that these choices are motivated by health, but the total dietary intake may not be healthy at all. Depending on the individually preferred foods, a patient may end up ingesting far too many supplemental vitamins and minerals from fortified bars and beverages. Individuals who are aware that their dietary intake is inadequate may also ingest excessive nutrients by self-prescribing multiple vitamin and mineral supplements in a misguided attempt to maintain health.

Substances That Interfere with Digestion or Absorption (Including Fiber, Fluids, and Foods Without Available Vitamins): Some individuals with eating disorders limit themselves to "filler" foods—bulky, nutrient-poor foods, such as rice cakes and bran cereal—that will provide a physical feeling of fullness with few calories. This type of eating can result in excessive fiber intake, inadequate nutrient intake, and limited absorption of nutrients that are ingested because of the binding action of fiber.

Convenience Foods, Preprepared Meals, and Foods Prepared Away from Home (Including Sodium, Energy Dense or High-Fat Foods and Beverages): During a binge episode, the nutrient quality of food is not usually a determining factor. In fact, chosen foods may be specifically less nutritious because of the patient's intention to purge after eating. Even for patients who do not purge, binge foods are often less nutritious and higher in fat and calories than patients normally "allow" themselves to eat.

Food in a Defined Period: Eating an excessive amount of food in a defined period is the definition of a binge. The word "binge" has many personal meanings for those who use it. Patients who tend to restrict their intake may consider any unplanned eating or even "normal" portions to be "bingeing." Clarify what constitutes a binge episode for each individual and avoid using the word binge when asking questions about food intake until you have confirmed that you understand each patient's personal definition.

Other Factors Associated with Excess Intake

Binge Eating Patterns: Finding out the times of day, types of food, and triggering situations related to an individual's binge eating will help you problem-solve and eventually provide advice to help change or stop the behavior. Keep in mind that patients with anorexia may struggle with or fear binge eating as much as patients with bulimia or binge eating disorder.

Change in Way Clothes Fit: Eating disorders are related to a disrupted sense of body size and shape, referred to as "body image distortion." For some individuals, changes (or lack of change) in the fit of clothes is the only way they can identify a change (or lack of change) in body size or weight. Patients may have clothing rules or routines, such as trying on a certain pair of jeans to see if they fit or refusing to try on certain sizes of clothing when shopping. Attempting to convince individuals that they are not the size that they imagine they are is rarely helpful in these situations. Body image can be so distorted that patients may insist that clothing they are wearing must be mismarked because it is impossible for them to fit in that size.

Highly Variable Calorie Intake: Many individuals with eating disorders will describe drastically varying eating patterns, often described as "good days" and "bad days." It is helpful to find out what constitutes the difference in intake and what triggers each type of day.

Assessment of Insufficient Intake

Carbohydrates and Fiber: The general label "carbs" has been applied to a variety of foods from whole grains to potatoes to fruit. If your patient reports limiting "carbs," clarify which foods are included in this category. Individuals who have developed an eating disorder after rapidly losing weight on such a diet will be reluctant to reincorporate carbs back into their lives.

Energy: Inadequate energy intake is not limited to individuals experiencing anorexia. Many individuals with bulimia or binge eating also consume inadequate energy when they are trying to avoid or compensate for a binge. Unfortunately this effort usually increases the likelihood of binge eating, convincing patients that they must try even harder to avoid all food.

Fluid: Avoiding fluid to reduce body weight is common in athletes required to weigh in; individuals who want to lose weight rapidly or fear that fluids cause bloating; or patients who want to avoid "feeling full."

Fat and Essential Fatty Acids: Possibly the most common type of nutrient avoided in eating disorders, dietary fat suffers from sharing its name with excess body fat. This leads many patients to attempt to eliminate all dietary fat from their intake, leaving them with limited food intake and poor absorption of fat-soluble nutrients. Adequate essential fatty acid intake is necessary for proper brain function and eating disorder recovery. Chronic fatty acid deficiency can also affect liver function. Increased liver enzymes should be monitored by a physician and often decrease over time as nutrition is restored.

Food (Including Supplements, Nutrients, Vitamins, and Minerals): Eating disorders often result in nutritional deficiencies because of food restrictions and rituals. Some individuals with eating disorders refuse to take any supplements to replenish nutrient stores, including a standard multivitamin–mineral pill because of their belief that supplements contain calories or that they will increase appetite.

Food or Foods from Specific Food Groups Caused by Gastrointestinal (GI) Symptoms: GI distress is commonly associated with eating after prolonged fasting, bingeing, purging, and any combination of these. The symptoms may be caused by the eating disorder, GI symptoms may predate the eating disorder, or the eating disorder may have developed as an individual eliminated different foods in an attempt to find the source of the problem. Individuals suffering with hemorrhoids or other conditions that make elimination painful may prefer not to eat at all. Additionally, athletes may avoid eating prior to competition to avoid needing to empty their bladder or bowels during the event.

Vitamin D and Sunlight Exposure: Once thought to be a concern primarily for individuals with inadequate dairy consumption or sunlight exposure, vitamin D deficiency is now recognized to be more common even in the general population. Individuals with restrictive eating patterns are particularly at risk.

Other Factors Associated with Insufficient Intake Anorexia: A lack of appetite can be caused by a variety of factors, including certain medications, depression, traumatic stress, and so on. Individuals with anorexia nervosa, however, may indeed experience hunger. Anorexia, the symptom, and anorexia, the disease, should not be assumed to go together.

Changes in Appetite or Taste: Zinc deficiency can lead to lack of sensitivity to taste and smell. Patients reporting changes in taste or reporting a recent propensity to salt, spice, or add other food flavorings, may be deficient in zinc, especially those who had been severely restricting their intake or following a vegetarian eating pattern. Note that overuse of condiments does not always indicate a zinc deficiency. It can also be a method of "ruining" food so that it is not edible.

Changes in Recent Food Intake and Recent Food Avoidance: Unfortunately, changes in food intake are not often recognized as the distress signal they so often are. When an individual suddenly changes his or her eating pattern, it is essential to attempt to determine what caused or instigated the change. Often something seemingly innocuous—a comment from a friend, an unexceptional doctor's appointment, a high school health class—can trigger an eating disorder in a susceptible individual. If identified early enough, an eating disorder may possibly be averted, and the root of the issue, whether anxiety, hurt feelings, or misinformation, can be addressed.

Forgetting to Eat: Not remembering to eat may be related to the hyperfocus associated with ADD, stress, heavy caffeine intake, or medication side effect. It may also be a fictitious explanation for restrictive eating.

Hunger: Our culture promotes the erroneous idea that "going hungry" is an effective weight-loss method. As a person becomes more starved, he or she thinks about food more often, which can lead to fears of overeating in patients with eating disorders. Patients with eating disorders may need frequent reassurance that eating when hungry does not cause excessive weight gain.

Lack of Interest in Food: One of the hallmarks of depression, an individual who genuinely lacks interest or desire to eat should be evaluated for depression by a mental health professional.

Lack of Strength or Stamina for Eating: A patient who is emaciated from starvation may require assistance or nutrition support in order to obtain adequate nutrition.

Mealtime Resistance or Refusal to Eat: Even an individual who voluntarily entered treatment may struggle to eat appropriately. If a patient is unable to eat independently, supervision at mealtimes and even nutrition support may be indicated.

Nausea or Early Satiety: Both nausea and early satiety are common during nutritional rehabilitation because of the disuse of the GI tract during starvation. For patients who are accustomed to eating only tiny amounts or used to inducing vomiting after eating, the sensation of food in the GI tract can provoke physical discomfort or pain along with mental distress. The physical discomfort should be referred to the primary physician, who may be able to recommend prescription or over-the-counter symptom management. It is important to convey to the patient that GI discomfort in many cases improves with regularity of eating and must not be allowed to impede nutritional rehabilitation.

Spitting Food Out: Chewing and spitting out food without swallowing ("sham eating") or swallowing and then regurgitating food are an effort to prevent digestion of food and therefore caloric intake. Chewing and spitting may be a learned behavior among athletes required to weigh in for their sport, post-bariatric surgery patients, and individuals with eating disorders, and may also be used to manage anxiety. This should be evaluated by a mental health professional.

Prolonged Mealtimes: Abnormally long mealtimes, reheating food during meals, cutting and mixing foods, and other specific rituals are different for each individual and will require problem solving on an individual basis. Setting time limits for meals and snacks may be appropriate.

Assessment of Intake Different from Recommended

Inappropriate Use of Food: Our culture unfortunately promotes many inappropriate uses of food, such as food as a reward, withholding of food as a punishment, forcing children to "clean their plates" to earn dessert, and so on. Adults with eating disorders may perpetuate inappropriate food rules from their childhoods and may create additional rules, all of which impair their ability to nourish themselves.

Inappropriate Choices of Food (Including Food Group and Nutrient Imbalance or a Limited Variety of Food): Inappropriate and unbalanced eating is common among individuals with eating disorders because of mistaken beliefs and fears about food.

Taking Medication (Over-the-Counter or Prescribed, Including Herbal, Botanical, or Dietary Supplements That Are Problematic or Inconsistent with Recommended Foods): You may encounter individuals who have become physically or psychologically dependent (or both) on over-the-counter or prescription medications, stimulants, laxatives, diet pills, and dietary supplements. Whether self-prescribed or recommended by a friend or pseudohealth professional, all such substances should be evaluated. Daily use or abuse of laxatives, stimulants, and prescription drugs should not be immediately discontinued except under a physician's care, as they may require a weaning protocol.

Protein or Other Supplementation: Excessive protein intake may be used in a misguided attempt to increase muscle mass or protect muscle mass during weight loss.

Assessment of Food and Nutrient Intolerance

Coughing or Choking with Eating: An evaluation of swallowing ability may be necessary to fully assess chewing or swallowing impairment. If coughing or choking is due to forcible feeding, this should be discouraged.

Diarrhea in Response to High Refined Carbohydrate Intake: This may occur inadvertently after a binge eating episode, or it can be used purposefully as a form of purging.

Feeling of Food "Getting Stuck" in the Throat: If individiuals have had bad experiences with food or traumatic incidents or injuries related to their mouths or faces, this can be a psychosomatic response that will require behavioral intervention and possibly medication to reduce anxiety. Medical causes, such as enlarged tonsils, swelling in the throat from an allergic reaction or procedure, and esophagitis from reflux should be evaluated and ruled out by a physician. A swallow study and intervention from a speech therapist may also provide information and recommendations.

Prolonged Chewing at Mealtime: See "Prolonged Mealtime" in the preceding section. Additionally, excessive chewing can be a misguided dieting method used to decrease appetite and caloric intake.

Assessment of Nutrition and Health Awareness

Awareness of Food or Calorie-Containing Beverages: Preoccupation with food and eating, in which a person relies excessively on nutrition terminology and fixates on the nutrient content of food, is often symptomatic of eating disorders and an effort to control fearful thoughts of weight gain and loss of control. Unfortunately, our culture promotes the hyperawareness of calories and certain nutrients in food and beverages, and this obsession can be admired and encouraged until it becomes excessive and impairs an individual's ability to function and eat normally.

Avoidance of Foods of Age-Appropriate Texture: This can result from tooth or mouth pain caused by malnutrition, self-injury, or ill-fitting dentures (particularly after weight loss), past bad experiences with food, or sensory issues. A swallow study and sensory evaluation may be helpful in recommending accommodations for texture modifications.

Avoidance of Foods or Food Groups (Including Fear of Foods or Dysfunctional Thoughts Regarding Food or Food Experiences): As with knowledge of caloric and nutrient content of foods, the ability to avoid certain foods and food groups is often looked on with admiration and called "willpower." But often it is also part of an eating disorder. There are certainly nonpathological reasons to avoid eating certain foods, but in cases where there is no allergy, intolerance, or special condition, an absolute rejection of all foods in a certain group is excessive and indicates a high level of anxiety that should be evaluated by a mental health professional.

Belief That Aging Can Be Slowed by Dietary Limitations: This is the hallmark belief of the "calorie restriction" movement. Not only do adherents to this methodology eat less than their daily energy needs, they also consume large quantities of dietary supplements. Although the focus of this eating style may not be weight loss, weight loss nevertheless results and is accompanied by preoccupation with health, longevity, or disease prevention. The term "orthorexia" is often used to describe this type of attempt to find the "most healthy" way of eating that ultimately leads to an eating disorder.[4] However, because orthorexia is not listed in the *Diagnostic and Statistical Manual of Mental Disorders, Fifth Edition* (*DSM-5*), anorexia nervosa or avoidant restrictive food intake behavior will be diagnosed.

**Chronic Dieting Behavior (Including Food Preoc-
cupation and Knowledge About Current Fad Diets):**
Although not recognized as a diagnosable eating disorder,
chronic dieting behavior and obsession with food can result
in nutrient deficiencies, psychological stress, impairment
in social functioning, excessive intake of bioactive substances, and other symptoms of eating disorders.

Cultural or Religious Practices That Limit Intake: Practices that limit intake should be evaluated in the context of
an individual's eating disorder, whether they predated the
eating disorder or are an attempt to justify it. Some mental
illnesses, such as schizophrenia and obsessive-compulsive
disorder, can include a pathological religious component.
Although it is not appropriate to discount a patient's religious beliefs, health concerns can override religious
customs, such as fasting, in many religions. Consultation
with a religious leader, either by the RDN, the patient, or
both, may be helpful. For a description of various religious and other eating practices, see "Appendix B: Guide
to Restrictive Eating Styles."

**Defensiveness, Hostility, or Resistance to Change (In-
cluding Denial of Hunger, Denial of Need for Food and
Nutrition-Related Changes, Frustration or Dissatis-
faction with Medical Nutrition Therapy [MNT] Recommendations, Lack of Appreciation of the Importance
of Making Recommended Nutrition-Related Changes,
Unwillingness or Disinterest in Applying Nutrition-
Related Recommendations, Verbalizing Unwillingness
or Disinterest in Learning):** Any and all of these are
potential responses to you and your assessment attempts if
an individual is not entering treatment by choice. Sometimes you will even encounter these behaviors in a patient
who is voluntarily in your care. Hostility can be an attempt
to "push you away" by a patient who is afraid of failing

or disappointing you, or it can be a symptom of a personality disorder, but either way it can impair your ability to
do your job. Discuss the situation with your supervisor
and the other members of the treatment team for advice on
how to approach the patient or whether it is more appropriate to work behind the scenes until the individual is more
approachable.

**Eating Alone, Feeling Embarrassed by the Amount of
Food Eaten, Eating Much More Rapidly Than Normal,
Eating Until Feeling Uncomfortably Full, Consuming Large Amounts of Food When Not Feeling Hungry,
Feeling a Sense of Lack of Control of Overeating During the Episode and Feeling Disgusted with Oneself,
Depressed, or Guilty After Overeating:** These are all
diagnostic criteria for binge eating disorder but can be
occasionally experienced by anyone. If these behaviors
are repeatedly experienced over time, then binge eating
disorder can be diagnosed. Regardless of the duration or
frequency of the episodes, nutrition counseling should
be accompanied by a mental health evaluation. Psychiatric evaluation may also be indicated if the binge eating is
related to depression, anxiety, traumatic stress, or another
mental health issue.

**Embarrassment or Anger at Need for Self-Monitoring
and Incomplete Self-Monitoring Records:** Embarrassment and anger may accompany a medical diagnosis even
if no one is at fault. It is important not to take this behavior
personally or to speak with your supervisor, support person, or other member of the treatment team if you do. Your
calm, nonjudgmental responses and willingness to work
with the patient, even without complete records, or to find
alternate methods to gather information are essential.

**Emotional Distress, Anxiety, or Frustration Surround-
ing Mealtimes:** These can be both a cause and consequence

of dysfunctional eating behaviors. Behavioral training from a mental health professional can help the patient learn to calm down before and during mealtimes, and a structured meal plan from you can free the patient from difficult mealtime decision making. If the distress, anxiety, and frustration are affecting the patient's family members, then counseling may be indicated for them as well. If family members are present during mealtime, then family counseling and individual counseling may be recommended, as well as coaching on appropriate mealtime behavior and expectations.

Food Faddism and Pica: Eating disorders may take the form of ingestion of nonfood substances intended to induce feelings of fullness (fiber tablets, chewing gum, cotton balls) or excessive quantities of foods reputed to cause weight loss (grapefruit, celery). Dangers range from GI distress to intestinal blockage. Pica can also take the form of compulsive ice chewing, a sign of iron-deficiency anemia. Excessive chewing of nonfood items (gum, pens, drinking straws, fingernails, and so forth) can also be a sign of anxiety and should be evaluated by a mental health professional.

Frustration over Lack of Control: Eating disorders are frustrating in many ways, most of all to the individuals attempting recovery. Healthy anger is directed at the eating disorder, at the duration of the recovery process, and at past behaviors and events. Unhealthy anger is directed at the treatment team or is internally focused. Your validation that these feelings are normal and your encouragement that improvement is on the horizon can be helpful, but the patient will also need to discuss these feelings with the mental health professional on the team. If frustration turns to thoughts of hopelessness and the patient indicates a wish to die, give up, or not be alive, this should be immediately reported to the physician or mental health professional on the team for direction. If you believe that a patient may be a danger to himself or herself or others and you are unable to speak with another team member, call 911 so that emergency medical personnel can transport the patient to a local emergency room.

Harmful Beliefs and Attitudes of Parents and Caregivers: See the "Inappropriate Use of Food" section. As you work with an individual to improve nutrition and eating behavior, include available family members and caregivers in your educational sessions. It can be difficult for patients to make needed changes without the support of family members they depend on.

Inflexibility with Food Selection: Professional opinions differ on whether individuals with eating disorders should be able to limit their food choices in recovery or should be forced to eat a balanced and varied diet. Ultimately this decision is up to you, based on your patient's situation, your clinical judgment, and, most significantly, the level of care in which you practice. In a residential or hospital facility you have complete control (in theory) of a person's intake, while in an outpatient setting you have none. Flexibility with food selection will take a long time for most patients; in the short term, adequacy of energy and nutrient intake is the priority. It may not be very important which foods are used to meet these needs. If a patient's preferences, however limited, can provide for his or her basic needs, it may be appropriate to work within these preferences until greater flexibility with food choices is possible.

Irrational Thoughts About Food's Effect on the Body (Weight Preoccupation): When an individual with an eating disorders step on a scale and see his or her weight, the past day's or week's intake immediately begin scrolling through his or her minds. The goal is to determine what was consumed that caused the weight change, whether up or down, and how to either fix it, undo it, or do it again. This leads to irrational thoughts about the grandiose effect a minute piece of food can have on body weight: "That peach had more than 60 calories, I knew it! That's why I gained weight!" As the RDN, your goal is not to remove this preoccupation with weight and food but to educate your patients that these thoughts are not realistic and to promote acceptance of normal fluctuations in body weight over time. Education about the weight of food and beverages during digestion, normal fluid shifts, and replenishment of nutrient stores can be helpful. Depending on your facility's protocol, decreasing the frequency of patient weighing or limiting the patient's access to his or her weight may be appropriate.

Previous Failures to Effectively Change Target Behavior: This may be the toughest mental obstacle your patient faces during recovery. If previous attempts at recovery have "failed," the patient may be feeling hopeless, helpless, discouraged, and so on. These feelings, unfortunately, add to the persistent underlying feelings of inadequacy that drive some eating disorders. Helping your patient identify things that have worked before, things he or she has learned in previous treatment settings, and pointing out even tiny steps of progress can help your patient learn to look at recovery in a more hopeful manner. If during an expression of hopelessness, your patient indicates a wish to die, give up, or not be alive, this should be immediately reported to the physician on the team.

Assessment of Food and Nutrient Knowledge and Skill

Food and Nutrition-Related Knowledge Deficit: Although an individual with an eating disorders may seem to have immediate command and recall of infinite bits of nutrition minutiae, he or she usually has little ability to apply it correctly. This is where you come in, teaching the *practice* of good nutrition, rather than simply the data.

Inability to Apply Food and Nutrition Information, Inability to Change Food or Activity Behavior, Inability to Maintain Weight or Regain Weight, Inability or Unwillingness to Select Food Consistent with Guidelines: It is a disappointing fact that all of your nutrition guidance and support alone may not be sufficient. There is only so much you can do, and even in the best of circumstances, some individuals simply cannot improve outside a treatment center or hospital. When, in the course of your assessment, you determine a patient is unwilling or unable to change, convey this information to the other team members to determine the appropriate treatment venue or level of care.

Lack of Ability to Prepare Meals and Uncertainty Regarding Foods to Prepare Based on Nutrition Prescription: The art of home meal preparation is experiencing a resurgence; however, many individuals need basic cooking training. You may also provide recipes, menu plans, or other structure to help eliminate the difficult decision-making problems some patients experience at mealtimes.

Assessment of Physical Activity

Decreased or Sedentary Activity Level: Many people have terrible memories of physical education in school, being picked last for teams, or having trouble exercising because of their size. The terms *exercise resistance* or *exercise avoidance* are used to describe why people who are physically able to exercise do not. Helping individuals overcome these barriers may be beneficial to weight-loss efforts and eating disorder recovery; however, behavioral counseling is indicated to help them move past bad experiences and look at physical activity in a different way. This of course does not apply to patients who have been instructed not to exercise by a medical provider.

Increased Physical Activity, Excessive Physical Activity (Ignoring Family or Job, Exercising Without Rest Days or While Injured or Sick), and Overtraining: Eating disorders often involve one or more attempts to override natural body signals, including hunger, pain, fatigue, and discomfort. Exercise can be used as a form of purging, a way to "earn" eating food, a mental escape from stress, a physical escape from an unhappy environment, and a pathway to admiration and a sense of accomplishment. Individuals restricted from exercise for medical reasons often become irritable, experiencing symptoms similar to substance withdrawal. They may feel compelled to stand instead of sit, fidget excessively, and secretly exercise, even under the covers while lying in bed. Patients with severe compulsivity to exercise or who are injured or have poor bone density may need to be monitored at all times to avoid further injury.

Assessment of Food Availability

Economic Constraints That Limit Availability of Appropriate Foods, Food Insecurity or Unwillingness to Use Available Resources, or Inability to Purchase and Transport Food to One's Home: For many years, eating disorders were wrongly considered diseases of the affluent. Now we understand that food insecurity is a direct risk factor for psychiatric disorder development. If a person is not purchasing, preparing, or bringing food into the home, then assess for financial distress, learning differences, geographical accessibility of markets, household pests, and ability to provide refrigeration. Arrange for financial assistance, transportation, or other services with the help of a social worker at your facility or through community programs in your area.

Assessment of Medications and Supplements

Insulin: Restricting insulin as a weight-loss tool is so common that it has its own name: diabulimia.[5] Eating disorders are twice as common among girls and women with insulin-dependent diabetes, and those with both diseases who misuse their insulin risk *triple* the rate of death from diabetes and its complications.[6] Any adolescent with insulin-dependent diabetes and any patient with a history of eating disorder who is newly diagnosed with diabetes, should be monitored for abnormal weight loss, ketone levels, and high blood glucose levels that may indicate dangerous manipulation of medication. (Note that eating disorders are not exclusive to type 1 diabetes. Recent research suggests approximately 15% of individuals with type 2 diabetes also meet criteria for an eating disorder.)[7]

Medication Associated with Weight Loss, Medications That Cause Anorexia, and Medications That Increase Energy Expenditure: Any medication that leads to weight loss, whether as its main purpose or as a side effect, has the potential to trigger an eating disorder in a susceptible individual. If the medication is temporary, then a fear of regaining lost weight can lead to restrictive eating after discontinuation of the medication. Chapter 4 contains a detailed list of medications associated with treatment of eating disorders.

Medication (Lipid Lowering): Some individuals are generally avoidant of medications and prefer to attempt lifestyle interventions instead. In the cases of high blood lipid levels, physicians may offer such a patient a timeline, such as 6 weeks or 3 months, to lower their levels via diet and exercise. This can promote inappropriate restriction of intake and excessive exercise that can trigger an eating disorder in susceptible individuals. Patients should instead be advised to use their prescribed medicine while they appropriately change behaviors to the point the medications are no longer needed. It is not uncommon to see elevated serum cholesterol levels in patients who restrict their eating. This type of high cholesterol will often be normalized with nutritional rehabilitation.

Medications Associated with Increased Appetite, Medications That Affect Appetite, Medications That Affect Resting Metabolic Rate (RMR), Medications That Impair Fluid Excretion, and Medications That Reduce Requirements or Impair Metabolism: Medication with the potential to increase appetite and weight can be frightening for anyone who fears weight gain. This can lead a patient to underuse or disregard prescribed medications or drastically restrict eating in an effort to counteract these effects.

Medications Requiring Nutrient Supplementation That Cannot Be Accomplished with Food Intake and Medications with Known Food-Medication Interactions: Whenever medications requiring nutrient supplementation or with food–drug interactions are prescribed, it is imperative to provide patients with education.

Misuse of Laxatives, Enemas, Diuretics, Stimulants, and Metabolic Enhancers: These substances are not only dangerous on their own, but can also provoke potentially dangerous interactions with prescribed medications. Reduction of these substances, in most cases, should be medically supervised.

Nutrition Assessment: Biochemical Data, Medical Tests, and Procedures

The results of an individual's laboratory tests will be helpful to his or her medical team, but may be of limited use in your nutrition assessment, as laboratory values are notoriously unreliable for assessing nutrient deficiencies in patients with eating disorders for a variety of reasons:[8]

- Their nutrition intake has, in most cases, declined over time, allowing metabolic and behavioral changes that result in energy and nutrient conservation.
- The individual's nutrient stores may be depleted, but most blood tests evaluate circulating nutrient levels, which may remain within normal limits.
- Dehydration, which often is found with an eating disorder, invalidates volume-dependent laboratory values, allowing them to appear normal until the patient achieves normal hydration status.
- Many patients with eating disorders take vitamin or mineral supplements or consume artificially fortified foods, such as energy bars, that mask their true long-term nutrition status.

It is generally accepted in the eating disorder treatment community that laboratory values within normal limits do not provide evidence of nutritional stability, yet patients, family members, and, at times, inexperienced health professionals can be deceived by normal laboratory test results. Laboratory values become more accurate and useful once nutritional rehabilitation has begun, but your nutrition assessment will likely be performed prior to nutritional rehabilitation. Regardless of the timing of your nutrition assessment, *abnormal* laboratory values should be taken very seriously, as they usually indicate *severe* and long-term nutritional deficiency.[2] Recommendations for nutrient supplementation based abnormal nutrient blood tests are found in Chapter 4 in the section, "Vitamin or Mineral Supplements." Table 2.1 provides additional information about laboratory tests that can add to your assessment of a patient with an eating disorder.

If available, the results of a dual energy x-ray absorptiometry scan (DEXA or DXA) show if the patient has normal (for age) or reduced bone density (osteopenia or osteoporosis). Depending on the results, the physician may limit physical activity because of bone fracture risk or may prescribe pharmaceutical intervention to replenish bone mass. Because bone formation relies on adequate circulating estrogen, amenorrhea can lead to bone porosity. Hormone replacement therapy in the form of oral contraceptives is often prescribed to women with eating disorders who are not menstruating, with the goal of protecting bone mass and preventing additional bone loss. Research, however, suggests that hormone replacement therapy is not effective at either.[2]

The biomedical section of your assessment may also include results of an electrocardiogram (ECG) or an echocardiogram. The ECG and echocardiogram reveal if the eating disorder has damaged the heart muscle and its function. The patient might experience decreased cardiac function as skipping beats, shortness of breath, heart pounding, chest pain during exercise, weakness, feeling light-headed, edema, or none of these. Based on the results, a physician may recommend limited physical activity, bed rest, or further cardiac monitoring. Any patient who has rapidly lost weight or has lost a significant percentage of body weight should be evaluated for cardiac stability by a cardiologist or other medical provider knowledgeable about eating disorders.[9]

Continued on next page.

Table 2.1 Laboratory Tests Related to Eating Disorders

Test	Relationship to eating disorders	Elevated in cases of	Decreased in cases of
Albumin	Indicator of nutrition status		Malnutrition Inflammation Shock Liver disease Crohn's disease Celiac disease
Amylase	Digestive enzyme produced mainly in salivary glands and pancreas. When either of these is inflamed, amylase escapes into the blood. Salivary isoamylase may be ordered when a patient is suspected of, but denies, vomiting to purge	Induced vomiting as a purging method Cholecystitis (gallbladder infection) Infection or obstruction of the salivary glands Intestinal obstruction Pancreatic or bile duct obstruction Perforated ulcer Tubal pregnancy (may be ruptured) Viral gastroenteritis Macroamylasemia	Low carbohydrate intake Damage to the pancreas Kidney disease Pancreatic cancer Toxemia of pregnancy

Table 2.1 (cont.) Laboratory Tests Related to Eating Disorders

Test	Relationship to eating disorders	Elevated in cases of	Decreased in cases of
Blood urea nitrogen (BUN)	Evaluates kidney function, which can be compromised in severe cases of eating disorders	Dehydration Catabolism of somatic protein as in starvation Excessive dietary protein intake Impaired kidney function Decreased blood flow to the kidneys due to congestive heart failure, shock, stress, recent heart attack, or severe burns Obstructed urine flow	Starvation Overhydration Liver disease
Calcium	Note: Blood calcium level does not reflect dietary calcium intake	Hyperparathyroidism Bone cancer	Malnutrition Alcoholism Magnesium deficiency Vitamin D deficiency Hypoparathyroidism

Continued on next page.

Table 2.1 (cont.) Laboratory Tests Related to Eating Disorders			
Test	Relationship to eating disorders	Elevated in cases of	Decreased in cases of
Complement C3	Sensitive indicator of nutrition status	Cancer Ulcerative colitis	Malnutrition Cirrhosis Hepatitis Lupus
Creatinine	Evaluates kidney function, which can be compromised in severe cases of eating disorders	Dehydration Muscle injury Impaired kidney function (can be caused by drug abuse), kidney stone Urinary tract obstruction Decreased blood flow to the kidneys due to shock, congestive heart failure, atherosclerosis, or complications of diabetes	Muscle wasting Pregnancy (due to increased blood volume)
Ferritin	Most sensitive indicator of iron status	Excessive iron supplementation Inflammation Liver disease Hemochromatosis (iron storage disease)	Inadequate dietary intake of iron

Continued on next page.

Table 2.1 (cont.) Laboratory Tests Related to Eating Disorders

Test	Relationship to eating disorders	Elevated in cases of	Decreased in cases of
Folate, vitamin B-9	Indicator of nutrition status; deficiency can cause altered mental status	Pernicious anemia Liver dysfunction	Malnutrition Alcohol abuse Celiac disease Crohn's disease Hemolytic anemia
Glucose	Indicator of bloodstream energy supply	Type 2 diabetes Type I diabetes (newly diagnosed or previously diagnosed but with inadequate insulin administration)	Acute malnutrition Too long without eating Inadequate carbohydrate intake Excess insulin administration
Hematocrit (HCT)	Indicator of nutrition status	Dehydration Polycythemia Blood doping Anabolic steroid use	Malnutrition Iron deficiency
Hemoglobin (Hgb)	Indicator of nutrition status	Dehydration	Malnutrition Iron deficiency
Human chorionic gonadotropin (hCG)	Pregnancy test	Pregnancy	

Continued on next page.

Table 2.1 (cont.) Laboratory Tests Related to Eating Disorders

Test	Relationship to eating disorders	Elevated in cases of	Decreased in cases of
Glycosylated Hemoglobin (HbA1c)	Measurement of blood glucose control over time	Poor glucose control Binge eating with type 2 diabetes Underuse of insulin with type 1 diabetes	
Iron	Indicator of nutrition status; deficiency can cause headache and fatigue, difficulty concentrating	Excessive iron supplementation Hemochromatosis	Inadequate dietary intake of iron Vegetarian dietary intake Heavy or long duration of menstruation Pregnancy Rapid growth in children
Lipase	An indicator of pancreas function	Pancreatitis and other pancreatic disease Kidney disease Salivary gland inflammation Bowel obstruction Peptic ulcer	Permanent pancreas damage

Continued on next page.

Table 2.1 (cont.) Laboratory Tests Related to Eating Disorders			
Test	Relationship to eating disorders	Elevated in cases of	Decreased in cases of
Liver function tests: alanine transaminase (ALT), alkaline phosphatase (ALP), aspartate transaminase (AST)	Evaluates liver function, which can be compromised in severe cases of eating disorders	Substance abuse (including alcohol, drugs, and steroids) Malnutrition Hepatitis	
Magnesium	Indicator of kidney and GI function	Dehydration Laxative abuse Excessive use of over-the-counter (OTC) antacids containing magnesium Hypothyroidism Addison's disease	Inadequate dietary intake of magnesium Diuretic abuse Laxative abuse Alcohol abuse Hypoparathyroidism Crohn's disease Irritable bowel disease (IBD) Celiac disease Surgery Burns Pregnancy

Continued on next page.

Table 2.1 (cont.) Laboratory Tests Related to Eating Disorders			
Test	Relationship to eating disorders	Elevated in cases of	Decreased in cases of
Mean corpuscular volume (MCV)	Indicator of nutrition status	Vitamin B-12 deficiency (macrocytic/ megaloblastic anemia) Alcoholism	Iron deficiency (microcytic anemia) Thalassemia
Phosphorus (P)	Indicator of nutrition status	Excessive supplementation	Refeeding syndrome Vomiting Laxative abuse Diuretic abuse Alcohol abuse Thyroid disease Untreated diabetes Kidney disease Malabsorption

Continued on next page.

Table 2.1 (cont.) Laboratory Tests Related to Eating Disorders			
Test	Relationship to eating disorders	Elevated in cases of	Decreased in cases of
Potassium (K)	Indicator of nutrition status	Dehydration due to inadequate fluid intake Untreated diabetes Excessive intake of foods high in vitamin K, excessive vitamin K supplementation Tissue injury Addison's disease Hypoaldosteronism Kidney failure Overuse of some medications, eg, nonsteroidal antiinflammatory drugs (NSAIDs), beta blockers, angiotensin-converting enzyme (ACE) inhibitors, and potassium-sparing diuretics	Refeeding syndrome Malnutrition Vomiting Dehydration due to diarrhea Acetaminophen overdose Hyperaldosteronism Abuse of diuretics Normal use of some medications, eg, corticosteroids; alpha- and beta-adrenergic agonists; some antibiotics, such as gentamicin and carbenicillin; and the antifungal agent amphotericin B

Continued on next page.

Table 2.1 (cont.) Laboratory Tests Related to Eating Disorders			
Test	Relationship to eating disorders	Elevated in cases of	Decreased in cases of
Red blood cell count (RBC)	Indicator of nutrition status	Dehydration	Iron deficiency
Thyroid-stimulating hormone (TSH)	Thyroid function may be abnormal due to or predating an eating disorder. Weight changes caused by thyroid dysfunction can complicate the diagnosis of eating disorders.	Starvation Hypothyroidism (acute or chronic) Pituitary tumor Inadequate administration of thyroid hormone when needed	Hyperthyroidism Excessive administration of thyroid hormone when needed Damage to the pituitary gland
Total protein	Indicator of nutrition status	Chronic infections HIV	Inadequate dietary intake of protein Celiac disease Irritable bowel disease Kidney disease Liver disease
Urine output	Indicator of fluid balance	Excessive fluid intake Psychogenic polydipsia Inadequate sodium intake	Dehydration (also evidenced by dark urine color)

Continued on next page.

Table 2.1 (cont.) Laboratory Tests Related to Eating Disorders

Test	Relationship to eating disorders	Elevated in cases of	Decreased in cases of
Urine specific gravity (USG)	Measurement of dehydration	Dehydration Diarrhea Urinary tract infection Excessive sweating	Renal failure Diabetes insipidus Excessive fluid intake
Vitamin B-12	Indicator of nutrition status; deficiency can cause altered mental status, contribute to depression	Serious underlying illness: liver disease, kidney failure, leukemia, polycythemia vera, hypereosinophilic syndrome	Pernicious anemia Vegetarian dietary intake (naturally occurs mainly in animal products) Post-bariatric surgery (especially Roux-en-Y gastric bypass [RYGP]) due to bypass of intrinsic factor secreted in stomach

Continued on next page.

Table 2.1 (cont.) Laboratory Tests Related to Eating Disorders

Test	Relationship to eating disorders	Elevated in cases of	Decreased in cases of
Zinc	Indicator of nutrition status; deficiency can cause altered sense of taste, difficulty gaining weight, and symptoms of depression	Excessive supplementation	Malnutrition Vegetarian dietary intake (naturally occurs mainly in animal products) High alcohol intake Chronic diarrhea Excessive exercise Sickle cell disease Chronic liver disease Post-bariatric surgery
25-Hydroxyvitamin D	Test for vitamin D deficiency	Excessive supplementation	Inadequate vitamin D intake Inadequate fatty acid intake Lack of exposure to sunlight Malabsorption Liver and kidney diseases Normal use of some medications, eg, phenytoin, phenobarbital, and rifampin

Nutrition Assessment: Anthropometric Measurements

If available at the time of your assessment, include the individual's:

- current weight,
- current height,
- current body mass index (BMI),
- recent weight change and usual body weight,
- highest and lowest body weights and under what circumstances, and
- body composition.

Nutrition Assessment: Nutrition-Focused Physical Findings

Physical symptoms of eating disorders vary from person to person, depending on the duration of the illness, type of eating and purging behaviors, and general physical well-being. Visible physical signs of eating disorders related to malnutrition and purging are listed in Box 2.2 (see pages 58–59), however, many individuals will not show any of these signs. Patients may present at or above a normal weight and may not show visible signs of malnutrition until well into the course of their illness. Therefore the information in Box 2.2 should be used as a guide, not as a diagnostic tool.

Nutrition Assessment: Patient History

In addition to gathering the patient's food and nutrition history, you will also gather information from the patient, family, treatment team, and medical chart about other aspects of the patient's medical and social history. Although you may not be personally asking the questions that gather this information, patient history may include some or all of the following topics. As you proceed, you may gather information that is new to the treatment team, and so confer with the patient on his or her preference about whether you or the patient will share that information with the team. Nutrition counseling alone will not be adequate to resolve all social and emotional issues. Nevertheless, as you ask about nutrition and related areas, you may identify other topics of importance. Chapter 6 details how to determine which areas fall under the realm of nutrition counseling and which should be referred to other disciplines or members of the team.

Patient history data categories and their relationship to eating disorders are described in detail in the following sections.

Social History

Abuse: A history of abuse can influence eating disorder treatment in many ways, as a patient may have feelings of low self-esteem, hopelessness, mistrust, or a dread of reaching a certain weight. Any time abuse is reported to you, refer to your treatment team or supervisor for guidance.

Avoidance of Social Events Where Food Is Served: A total avoidance of food-related events may indicate the presence of a social anxiety disorder in addition to the eating disorder. If social events are required for employment or other reasons, problem-solving these events will be an important part of your nutrition counseling strategy.

Change in Living Environment and Independence: Moving to a new environment can trigger an eating disorder in a susceptive individual.

Substance Abuse: Substance abuse includes laxatives, diuretics, diet pills, and steroids, in addition to street drugs, prescription drugs, and stimulants. Some individuals may

Box 2.2 Nutrition-focused Physical Findings

Head and Neck

Ketone smell on breath due to inadequate carbohydrate intake

Oral lesions due to erosion by stomach acid during vomiting

Dry or cracked lips due to vitamin deficiency or dehydration

Enlarged parotid glands due to vomiting

Damaged teeth due to erosion by stomach acid during vomiting

Hair loss due to malnutrition

Lanugo hair on face due to malnutrition, low body temperature

Occipital wasting due to muscle wasting

Broken blood vessel in eye due to vomiting

Gastrointestinal

Constipation, abdominal distension due to binge eating, induced vomiting, delayed gastric emptying, rebound constipation after laxative abuse, inadequate fluid intake, excessive fluid intake

Blood visible in emesis due to esophageal erosion or broken blood vessels from repeated vomiting

Blood visible in stool due to constipation leading to hemorrhoids, misuse of laxatives

Reflux (gastroesophageal reflux disease [GERD]) may be preexisting or may be due to frequent regurgitation; may be related to binge eating, abdominal adiposity, anxiety

Neurologic

Impaired concentration, neurological changes (eg, depressed, irritable mood) due to malnutrition and inadequate intake of carbohydrates, essential fatty acids, B vitamins, and vitamin D

Cardiovascular

Arrhythmias due to starvation, misuse of ipecac, electrolyte imbalance caused by induced vomiting, excessive exercise

Dizziness, shortness of breath, diminished cardiac function due to muscle wasting, inadequate fluid intake, orthostatic hypotension, bradycardia, excessive exercise

Continued on next page.

Box 2.2 (cont.) Nutrition-focused Physical Findings

Extremities and Musculoskeletal

Arthralgia due to malnutrition

Bone fragility due to malnutrition leading to amenorrhea and decreased bone formation, inadequate calcium and vitamin D intake, inadequate dietary calcium intake

Decreased body fat due to starvation

Acrocyanosis of hands and feet due to malnutrition, reduced circulation and cardiac function, reduced body temperature

Frequent and prolonged injuries due to malnutrition, excessive exercise, refusal to rest or recuperate

Decreased muscle mass due to starvation

Delayed capillary refill

Russell's sign (scars, scabs on knuckles) due to using fingers to induce vomiting

Skin

Peripheral edema due to malnutrition

Dry skin due to malnutrition

Acanthosis nigricans due to insulin resistance

Vital Signs

Hypotension due to starvation

Orthostatic hypotension due to dehydration

Bradycardia due to starvation, decreased cardiac function, cardiac muscle wasting

Decreased temperature due to metabolic conservation effects of starvation regulated by hypothalamus turn to cocaine, heroin, methamphetamine, or prescription stimulants in an effort to control their weight. Co-occurring substance abuse is very common in eating disorders and should be addressed at the same time as the eating disorder to help the patient avoid simply switching back and forth.[10]

Lack of Developmental Readiness: Independent eating may not be age appropriate for children with eating disorders. Your time may be better spent with parents or other caregivers, providing guidelines for feeding, including appropriate portion sizes, food choices, timing of meals and snacks, and mealtime behavior.

Lack of Funds for Purchase of Appropriate Foods: For many years, eating disorders were wrongly considered diseases of the affluent. Now we understand that food insecurity is a direct risk factor for eating disorder development. If a patient is not purchasing, preparing, or bringing food into the home, assess for financial distress, learning differences, geographical accessibility of markets, household pests, and ability to provide refrigeration. Arrange for financial assistance, transportation, or other services with the help of a social worker at your facility or through community programs in your area.

Lack of Suitable Support System to Access Food: Children and teens who do not have their own source of income or transportation rely on their caregivers for food procurement and preparation. Because of economics and other family situations, many children and teens spend their after-school time alone, fending for themselves. Children with eating disorders are unlikely to go out of their way to eat, especially without supervision. Education and guidance for the caregivers and the patient (eg, prepare food ahead of time for the child to snack on, show child how to safely use the microwave, and so forth) can be beneficial in these situations.

Recent Lifestyle Changes: A divorce, death, marriage, move, new school, empty nest, or more than one of these can be overwhelming, especially if there are mixed feelings, confusion, and difficult adjustments. Often such changes prompt a desire for weight loss, even if unneeded, and can trigger an eating disorder. Although you can help individuals manage their eating during this time, underlying stressors should be referred to mental health professionals on the team.

New Medical Diagnosis or Change in Condition: It is easy to see how a new diagnosis, especially one that requires a special diet or change in eating habits, could trigger an eating disorder. For someone with an existing eating disorder, a new diagnosis or change in condition can be especially discouraging, leading him or her to think that recovery is unattainable or "not worth it."

Personal and Family History

History of Childhood Obesity: Many underweight eating disorder patients report a history of overweight or perceived overweight in childhood. This strongly affects their beliefs about themselves and their abilities to maintain a "normal" weight without extreme measures. Asking additional questions about why the individual thinks he or she was overweight ("I watched too much television"; "I ate too many snacks") in the past may help gather more information about current food fears and rituals.

History of Familial Obesity: Individuals whose parents were or are obese may excessively restrict their eating in a misguided effort to prevent their own obesity. Eating disorders may develop, resulting in weight loss for some, and overweight for others, which is the very condition they had hoped to avoid. If overweight family members also experienced chronic dieting or binge eating, your patient may never have observed any role models who were truly healthy eaters.

History of Eating Disorders, Depression, Obsessive Compulsive Disorders, or Anxiety Disorders: Family psychiatric history, including addictions, is related to eating disorders. Although the exact genetic and neurochemical links are not yet fully understood, this information may provide a level of comfort to patients and family members, helping them realize that their eating disorder is not their "fault."

History of Hyperlipidemia, Atherosclerosis, or Pancreatitis: Family history of heart disease and related factors, especially if it was implicated in the early death of one or more relatives, leads many individuals to modify their eating. Those with a predisposition to eating disorders may take this to an extreme, such as attempting to reduce their fat intake to zero, or other abnormal and unhealthy measures. Ironically, anorexia can cause cholesterol levels to increase, because the effects of starvation and low-fat, high-carbohydrate eating can lead to increased triglyceride levels. In the mind of someone with an eating disorder, these results can prove that even further restrictions are necessary.

History of Inability to Lose Weight Through Conventional Intervention: Unsuccessful attempts to lose weight can be very discouraging, especially when your patient is "doing everything right." The frustration can lead to harmful weight-loss attempts, triggering an eating disorder. In some of these cases, the patient will never succeed with weight loss because he or she is fighting an undiagnosed endocrine disorder. When a patient describes *gaining* weight while dieting, rapid weight loss or weight gain without a change in eating, abnormal appetite or cravings surrounding menstruation, or lack of weight loss even though eating minimally and exercising, an endocrine consult is in order. Hormone abnormalities are not rare in the eating disorder population, but they do go undiagnosed. Diabetes, polycystic ovary disease (PCOS), hyper- and hypothyroidism, Cushing syndrome, and others can all interfere with body weight regulation. Appropriate diagnosis by an endocrinologist or other medical doctor and treatment are essential.

Medical and Health History

Alcoholism: Alcohol dependence and abuse commonly co-occur with eating disorders. If an individual with an eating disorder also abuses alcohol, both conditions require treatment concurrently so that the patient does not simply switch back and forth.

Anxiety Disorder: Anxiety is a common co-occurring disorder with eating disorders. Appropriate treatment, usually a combination of medication and counseling, is essential, as eating disorder recovery requires the patient to participate in anxiety-provoking behaviors, such as eating more than he or she desires or eating feared foods. The neurochemical link between eating disorders and anxiety disorders is not yet fully understood; however, eating disorder behaviors may function as one way of reducing anxiety.

Binge Eating: Binge eating is obviously a problem for a patient with binge eating disorder or bulimia, but it can also plague someone with anorexia.

Breast Surgery: Individuals undergo breast augmentation for a variety of reasons, but those with severely distorted body image or body dysmorphic disorder may choose repeated cosmetic surgery. Breast augmentation can also conceal the skeletal frame of a woman with anorexia whose own breast tissue is minimal.

Cardiovascular Disease, Hyperlipidemia, Hypertriglyceridemia, Hypertension, and Metabolic Syndrome: A diagnosis of cardiovascular disease usually is delivered together with recommendations to decrease intake of fat and saturated fat, increase physical activity, and so on. In some cases, an effort to make dietary changes because of fear can lead to an eating disorder. In others, a patient who has concealed his or her eating disorder from the physician can use the diagnosis as an excuse to perpetuate eating disorder behaviors, such as inadequate intake and excessive exercise. Discuss with the patient the importance of disclosing his or her eating disorder diagnosis with the doctor, and advocate with the doctor for a collaborative treatment plan to treat the eating disorder and cardiovascular disease concurrently.

Celiac Disease, Crohn's Disease, Diverticulitis, Inflammatory Bowel Disease, Irritable Bowel Syndrome, Lactase Deficiency, Malabsorption, Maldigestion, Polyps in the Colon, and Prolapsing Hemorrhoids: Any diagnosis that causes GI pain or requires a drastic change in eating habits can trigger eating disorders in susceptible individuals. Additionally, if prior to diagnosis, a patient has experienced unexplained GI distress, he or she may have unnecessarily eliminated many foods attempting to find the source of the problem.

Chronic Fatigue Syndrome: The exact connection between chronic fatigue syndrome and eating disorders is unknown, but they do co-occur in some cases.

Cleft Lip or Palate and Oral Soft Tissue Infection: As with anything that impairs the eating experience or makes it unpleasant or uncomfortable, a cleft lip and palate, even once repaired, can trigger food restriction and eating disorders. Any kind of mouth infection, pain, sore, or surgery can do the same. Oral sores can be caused by repeated vomiting and can become infected.

Cognitive or Emotional Impairment: Anything that leads an individual to feel "different," "not good enough," or not accepted by peers can lead to an attempt to lose weight, whether warranted or not, in order to "fit in." This of course can trigger an eating disorder.

Constipation: A common symptom of GI disuse (caused by inadequate intake, "rebound" constipation from laxative abuse, or vomiting), constipation lasting more than a few days should be evaluated by a physician. As a patient becomes more and more impacted, he or she generally becomes less and less willing to continue following a meal plan, in which case a nonstimulant laxative or other medication may be prescribed. If a patient has a history of laxative abuse, a supportive family member may be willing to hold the medication and distribute it as recommended by the physician.

Cushing Syndrome: A primary symptom is weight gain, which can trigger, or be mistaken for, an eating disorder.

Cystic Fibrosis and Diabetes: The stress of a chronic illness, especially one that requires extra focus on food, eating, and medication at mealtimes, can trigger rebellion in the form of refusing to follow recommendations. Missing school because of medical appointments, trips to the nurse's office, and other facets of these illnesses that lead a child or teen to "feel different" can also be triggers for eating disorders. Skipping medications in order to manipulate weight can give a false sense of control in a frustrating situation. Unfortunately the consequences can be dire. Both types 1 and 2 diabetes are associated with eating disorders and with high risk of complications.[5-7]

Dementia: Eating disorders in the elderly population have not been studied to the extent of eating disorders in adolescence, yet it is clear that many issues coexist between eating disorders and the aging process.

Depression: Depression is another commonly co-occurring disorder with eating disorders. Once again the connections are not clear, but inadequate intake can lead to neurochemical disruption and depression, and depression can cause a lack of interest in food. Depression related to eating disorders may improve with nutritional rehabilitation, but it should also be evaluated and treated separately, usually with medication and counseling, if it persists.

Fatigue: This, of course, can be a result of malnutrition. Fatigue can also impair a person's ability and desire to obtain and prepare food, thereby perpetuating or worsening malnutrition.

Foodborne Illness: Avoiding a food that once gave you food poisoning seems like a perfectly normal reaction. An eating disorder, however, may lead someone to avoid a whole food group, all food not personally prepared, or all foods entirely because of fear of food contamination. This is especially the case for patients who also have an anxiety or obsessive-compulsive disorder.

Fractures (Stress): Stress fractures are common in eating disorder patients who exercise against medical advice, exercise excessively, or have osteoporosis caused by malnutrition.

Headache: Because of malnutrition and dehydration, headaches are common.

Hyperthyroidism and Hypothyroidism: Permanent endocrine dysfunction is occasionally the result of severe malnutrition. When people with eating disorders are given medicine that increases their metabolic rate, such as levothyroxine (Synthroid), it can be very tempting to use it improperly to promote weight loss.

Hypoglycemia: Usually a result of inappropriate spacing between meals, hypoglycemia may persist after recovery, or it may resolve with nutritional rehabilitation.

Illness (Recent): Involuntary weight loss, such as that caused by an illness, can trigger an eating disorder in a susceptible person. Once the weight is lost, the patient may not want to gain it back, leading to restrictive eating. In other cases, an illness that requires someone to leave school or work or miss a vacation or other event can lead to depression and possibly an eating disorder.

Mental Illness: Bipolar disorder, schizophrenia, oppositional defiant disorder, depression, anxiety, ADD, and obsessive-compulsive disorder all commonly co-occur with eating disorders. If untreated, they may interfere with eating disorder treatment. Some of the medications widely used to treat these disorders affect appetite and weight, in which case an eating disorder can result if the patient uses extreme measures to counteract unwanted weight gain.

Multiple Sclerosis: In the category of life-changing major illness is multiple sclerosis, which can result in depression and manipulation of food in an effort to find control.

Obesity and Overweight: Unfortunately, many eating disorders go undiagnosed because of a pervasive misconception that eating disorders are only associated with underweight individuals. Binge eating disorder may be more common than anorexia and bulimia nervosa combined, a recognition that hopefully will help the medical community avoid using weight as the only criteria for identifying eating disorders.

Personality Disorder: Narcissistic, borderline, passive-aggressive, avoidant, and obsessive-compulsive personality disorders can co-occur with eating disorders.[11] If your patient has been identified as having a personality disorder, speak with the mental health professional on the team for advice on how to proceed with the patient and how to learn about the condition. Progress may be slower than even the usual slow progress of eating disorder treatment, and you may experience feelings that surprise you, such as hopelessness, helplessness, frustration, irritation, or inadequacy. These are common reactions to working with a patient with severe personality issues, and it is important that you are able to view them as functions of the disorder, not evidence that you are ineffective as an RDN. Dialectical behavioral therapy can be a beneficial treatment for borderline personality disorder.

Polycystic Ovary Disease: PCOS, also known as "chronic anovulation," results from insulin resistance but manifests as difficulty maintaining a normal weight, carbohydrate and sweet cravings, and irregular menstruation.[12] Women with PCOS are often not aware of their condition, so they drastically restrict their dietary intake in an effort to lose or maintain weight, potentially triggering an eating disorder. Although cystic ovaries (not the same as an ovarian cyst) are visible via a sonogram, some women with PCOS do not actually manifest the very symptom the condition is named for. Instead, they will have abnormal blood tests, specifically their reproductive hormones and their insulin-to-glucose ratio. Severe acne, abnormal facial or body hair (distinct from lanugo), acanthosis, and skin tags can also be signs of PCOS. Treatment for PCOS will be needed to assist the patient in eating disorder recovery.

Premenstrual Syndrome: For many women, the days before and during menstruation are accompanied by mood changes and food cravings. Educate your patient about the influence of reproductive hormones and the normalcy of these cravings and physical symptoms, such as bloating, to help diminish the shame associated with perceived weight gain and lack of control of eating. Medical management may be available if symptoms are severe.

Tardive Dyskinesia: A side effect of some antipsychotic medications results in involuntary movements. Depending on what part of the body is affected, these movements can interfere with eating or can increase energy needs above normal.

Tremors: Tremors can be a sign of withdrawal from alcohol, as well as other disorders. Ensure that the medical provider is aware of the tremors.

Other Issues

Abdominal Cramping, Abdominal Pain, Bloating, Constipation, Diarrhea, Epigastric Pain, Flatulence, Gastrointestinal Disturbances, Nausea, and Self-Induced Vomiting: As noted earlier, these are commonly associated with eating after long periods of starvation or purging and may require medical evaluation and symptom management.

Amenorrhea: Missing three menstrual periods in a row is no longer a criterion of diagnosis of anorexia nervosa. It can result from malnutrition as well as underlying hormonal disorders.

Anorexia: A lack of appetite (anorexia the symptom) can be caused by a variety of factors, including certain medications, medical conditions, and depression. Individuals with anorexia nervosa, however, may or may not experience hunger.

Dizziness and Unexplained Falls: Inadequate nutrition and especially dehydration can cause orthostatic changes, that is, an inadequate blood pressure response when moving to standing up from a seated position. Individuals experiencing dizziness on standing, fainting, or "blacking out" should be evaluated medically and advised on appropriate physical activities (or restrictions) needed to prevent injury. Bed rest, sitting for a few minutes on the side of the bed before standing, adequate fluid intake, salt intake, electrolyte-containing beverages, baths instead of showers, or restriction from driving a car and exercising are examples of recommendations that may be appropriate.

Hunger or Use of Alcohol or Drugs That Reduce Hunger: These may include over-the-counter or prescription diet pills, illegal drugs, nicotine, and caffeinated beverages. If a patient is physically or psychologically dependent on one or more of these substances, a weaning protocol may be required under medical supervision.

Muscle Weakness, Fatigue, Cardiac Arrhythmia, Dehydration, Electrolyte Imbalance, and Shortness of Breath: These can result from malnutrition and require medical evaluation.

Report of Always Feeling Cold: Also called cold intolerance, this is a result of physiological adaptation to starvation; body temperature decreases and adipose tissue normally used to produce heat and insulate the core is used for energy.

Medical Treatments or Procedures

Chemotherapy with Oral Side Effects, Radiation Therapy, or Surgery: Cancer is a life-altering diagnosis that can trigger an eating disorder, as can involuntary weight loss caused by illness or medications. Oral or GI side effects of treatment, including pain medication, potentially multiply this effect.

Gastric Bypass: As surgeries for the purpose of weight loss have become more common, the number of post-surgery patients in treatment for eating disorders continues to rise. It may be impossible to distinguish which came first: the eating disorder or the weight problem, the weight problem or the depression, the eating disorder or the post-surgical weight loss, the eating disorder or the post-surgery complications, the eating disorder or the post-surgical weight loss and regain, and so forth. Gastric bypass or other weight-loss surgery should be considered a risk factor for eating disorders.

Knee Surgery: Knee injury is one of the most common career-ending injuries for high-level athletes. Athletes at the competitive and elite levels have dedicated much or most of their lives to their sport, and the inability to continue to compete can be devastating to their identity and self-esteem. The potential for (and fear of) weight gain if the patient continues to eat at the same high-energy level needed during training can trigger an eating disorder in a susceptible individual. Patients in this situation require nutrition counseling regarding their nutrient and energy needs for healing and then on an ongoing basis if their level of physical activity will be drastically different post-surgery.

Oral Surgery: For obvious reasons, oral surgery can impair the ability and desire to eat and may cause pain on chewing, swallowing, or both. Involuntary weight loss caused by an inability to eat normally can trigger an eating disorder or may be welcomed by an individual with an eating disorder.

Ostomy: The discomfort of an ostomy, especially a new ostomy, can reduce a patient's willingness to eat. Also, an ostomy can be the unfortunate result of long-term or severe abuse of laxatives.

References

1. Kellogg M. *Counseling Tips for Nutrition Therapists: Practice Workbook*. Vol 2. Philadelphia, PA: Kg Press; 2009.

2. Yager J, Devlin MJ, Halmi KA, et al. *Practice Guideline for the Treatment of Patients with Eating Disorders*. 3rd ed. Arlington, VA: American Psychiatric Association; 2006.

3. Setnick J. *The Eating Disorders Clinical Pocket Guide: Quick Reference for Healthcare Providers*. Dallas, TX: Snack Time Press; 2005.

4. Koven NS, Abry AW. The clinical basis of orthorexia nervosa: emerging perspectives. *Neuropsychiatr Dis Treat*. 2015;11:385-394.

5. Mathieu J. What is diabulimia? *J Am Diet Assoc*. 2008;108(5): 769-770.

6. Goebel-Fabbri AE, Fikkan J, Franko DL, et al. Insulin restriction and associated morbidity and mortality in women with type 1 diabetes. *Diabetes Care*. 2008;31:415-419.

7. Nicolau J, Simo R, Sanchis P, et al. Eating disorders are frequent among type 2 diabetic patients and are associated with worse metabolic and psychological outcomes: results from a cross-sectional study in primary and secondary care settings. *Acta Diabetol*. 2015; 52(6):1037-1044.

8. Setnick J. Micronutrient deficiencies and supplementation in anorexia and bulimia nervosa: a review of literature. *Nutr Clin Pract*. 2010;25(2):137-142.

9. Gilbert SD, Commerford MC. *The Unofficial Guide to Managing Eating Disorders*. Foster City, VA: IDG Books Worldwide; 2000.

10. Helfman BL, Dennis AB. Understanding the complex relationship between eating disorders and substance use disorders. *Renfrew Perspect*. 2010;(Winter):2-4.

11. Sansone RA, Sansone LA. Personality disorders as risk factors for eating disorders: clinical implications. *Nutr Clin Pract.* 2010;25(2):116-121.

12. Grassi A. *The Dietitian's Guide to Polycystic Ovary Syndrome (PCOS).* Philadelphia, PA: Luca Publishing; 2007.

Chapter 3

Nutrition Diagnosis for Eating Disorders

The Nutrition Care Process organizes nutrition diagnoses into three different groups: Intake, Clinical, and Behavioral-Environmental. The most pertinent and urgent nutrition-related problem should be chosen for the nutrition diagnosis and phrased in problem, etiology, and signs and symptoms (PES) format:

> [Nutrition diagnosis term (problem)] related to
> [etiology] as evidenced by [signs and symptoms].

Tables 3.1 through 3.3 provide sample Nutrition Diagnoses for the different eating disorder diagnoses and for different presenting problems that you may observe. These examples do not cover all of the possibilities and patients you may encounter, so use them as a guide for your own patient-specific PES statements.

Although there may be many nutrition-related issues for each individual with an eating disorder, remember to prioritize the most pertinent and urgent nutrition-related problem(s) in your initial nutrition diagnosis. Note that the diagnosis "harmful beliefs/attitudes about food and nutrition" may not be used as a nutrition diagnosis for someone with an eating disorder but may be used in the evidence portion of the statement.

Table 3.1 Sample Nutrition Diagnoses for Anorexia Nervosa and Avoidant Restrictive Food Intake Disorder

Problem (P)	Etiology (E) (choose one)	Signs/Symptoms (S) (choose one or more)
Inadequate energy intake	Disordered eating Diagnosis of anorexia nervosa (AN) or avoidant restrictive food intake disorder (ARFID) Increased energy needs due to hypermetabolism Lack of interest in food due to depression Obsessive desire to lose weight Harmful beliefs about eating Excessive physical activity	Failure to maintain appropriate weight Depleted adipose and somatic protein stores Bradycardia (heart rate < 60 beats per minute) Amenorrhea Fear of food Laboratory values reflecting malnutrition Hypoglycemia Irrational beliefs about the effects of food on the body Restriction or refusal of food or energy-dense food
Excessive fluid intake	Disordered eating Diagnosis of AN or ARFID Harmful beliefs about eating	Water or noncaloric beverage intake exceeding estimated needs Hyponatremia
Excessive intake of caffeine or other dietary stimulants	Disordered eating Diagnosis of AN Harmful beliefs about eating	Frequent or excessive intake of coffee or tea, caffeinated sodas, "energy" drinks or caffeine pills

Continued on next page.

Table 3.1 (cont.) Sample Nutrition Diagnoses for Anorexia Nervosa and Avoidant Restrictive Food Intake Disorder

Problem (P)	Etiology (E) (choose one)	Signs/Symptoms (S) (choose one or more)
Excessive intake of dietary fiber	Disordered eating Diagnosis of AN Harmful beliefs about eating	Constipation or diarrhea, flatulence or abdominal distension related to excessive intake of high-fiber foods or fiber supplements
Inadequate vitamin/mineral intake (specify individual vitamins and minerals if applicable)	Increased nutrient needs due to prolonged catabolism Disordered eating Diagnosis of AN or ARFID Harmful beliefs about eating	Abnormal laboratory values (specify) Physical findings (specify) Dietary intake inadequate compared with estimated needs
Underweight	Disordered eating Excessive physical activity Diagnosis of AN or ARFID Harmful beliefs about eating	Decreased skin-fold thickness and midarm muscle circumference Body mass index (BMI) < 18.5 Muscle wasting Inadequate intake of food compared to estimated needs
Inadequate fat intake	Disordered eating Diagnosis of AN or ARFID Harmful beliefs about eating	Avoidance of foods containing fats Irrational beliefs about the effects of fats on the body Dermatitis (scaly skin) consistent with essential fatty acid deficiency

Continued on next page.

Table 3.1 (cont.) Sample Nutrition Diagnoses for Anorexia Nervosa and Avoidant Restrictive Food Intake Disorder

Problem (P)	Etiology (E) (choose one)	Signs/Symptoms (S) (choose one or more)
Inadequate protein intake	Disordered eating Diagnosis of AN or ARFID Food- and nutrition-related knowledge deficit (especially if patient is vegetarian or vegan) Harmful beliefs about eating Edema Skin breakdown	Insufficient intake of protein sources compared with estimated needs Prolonged adherence to a very-low-protein weight-loss diet, vegetarian or vegan diet or unbalanced, restrictive diet Laboratory values reflecting low protein intake
Inadequate carbohydrate intake	Disordered eating Diagnosis of AN or ARFID Harmful beliefs about eating	Avoidance of high-carbohydrate foods Irrational beliefs about the effects of carbohydrates on the body Insufficient intake of carbohydrate compared with estimated needs Hypoglycemia Low serum amylase
Inadequate fluid intake	Excessive physical activity Disordered eating ARFID Harmful beliefs about drinking fluids	Acute weight loss Insufficient intake of fluids compared with estimated needs Elevated blood urea nitrogen (BUN) level Elevated sodium (Na) level Plasma or serum osmolality > 290 mOsm/kg

Continued on next page.

Table 3.1 (cont.) Sample Nutrition Diagnoses for Anorexia Nervosa and Avoidant Restrictive Food Intake Disorder		
Problem (P)	Etiology (E) (choose one)	Signs/Symptoms (S) (choose one or more)
Disordered eating pattern	Obsessive desire to lose weight Undue influence of weight on self-esteem	Abnormal laboratory values (specify) Irrational beliefs about the effects of food on the body Intake reflecting an imbalance of food groups Avoidance of food or food groups (specify) Food rituals (specify) Lengthy period of time without eating
Excessive exercise	Inability to rest and recuperate as advised by physician Diagnosis of AN Obsessive desire to lose weight Harmful beliefs about food Fatigue despite adequate energy intake and duration of sleep	Weight loss Depleted adipose and somatic protein stores Stress fracture or other overuse injury Exercising when sick, injured, or in defiance of medical recommendations Neglect of family, work, or other responsibilities to exercise Exercise exceeding levels needed to improve health or athletic performance Exercise specifically in response to foods eaten

Table 3.2 Sample Nutrition Diagnoses for Bulimia Nervosa or Purging Disorder

Problem (P)	Etiology (E) (choose one)	Signs/Symptoms (S) (choose one or more)
Inadequate energy intake	Disordered eating Diagnosis of bulimia nervosa (BN) or purging disorder (PD) Obsessive desire to lose weight Excessive physical activity	Fear of food Self-induced vomiting (purging) Refusal of food due to fear of purging Oligomenorrhea or amenorrhea Irrational beliefs about the effects of food on the body Weight loss Restriction or refusal of energy-dense food
Excessive energy intake Excessive oral food/ beverage intake	Disordered eating Diagnosis of BN Resolution of prior hypermetabolism without reduction in intake	Body fat > 32% (women) or > 25% (men) BMI > 25 (adults) or > 95th percentile Weight gain Intake of high caloric density or large portions of food/ beverages Binge eating Emotional eating
Excessive fluid intake	Disordered eating Diagnosis of BN or PD Harmful beliefs about eating	Water or noncaloric beverage intake exceeding estimated needs Hyponatremia Clear urine
Excessive intake of caffeine or other dietary stimulants	Disordered eating Diagnosis of BN Harmful beliefs about eating	Frequent or excessive intake of coffee or tea, caffeinated sodas, energy drinks, or caffeine pills

Continued on next page.

Table 3.2 (cont.) Sample Nutrition Diagnoses for Bulimia Nervosa (BN) or Purging Disorder (PD)

Problem (P)	Etiology (E) (choose one)	Signs/Symptoms (S) (choose one or more)
Excessive intake of dietary fiber	Disordered eating Diagnosis of BN Harmful beliefs about eating	Constipation or diarrhea, flatulence or abdominal distension related to excessive intake of high-fiber foods or fiber supplements
Inadequate vitamin/ mineral intake (specify individual vitamins or minerals if applicable)	Disordered eating Diagnosis of BN Harmful beliefs about eating	Abnormal laboratory values (specify) Physical findings (specify) Purging Dietary intake inadequate compared with estimated needs
Inadequate fat intake	Disordered eating Diagnosis of BN Harmful beliefs about eating	Avoidance of foods containing fats Irrational beliefs about the effects of fats on the body Purging Dermatitis (scaly skin) consistent with essential fatty acid deficiency
Inadequate protein intake	Disordered eating Diagnosis of BN Food- and nutrition-related knowledge deficit (especially if patient is vegetarian or vegan) Harmful beliefs about eating	Insufficient intake of protein sources compared with estimated needs Purging Laboratory values reflecting low protein intake Edema Skin breakdown

Continued on next page.

Table 3.2 (cont.) Sample Nutrition Diagnoses for Bulimia Nervosa (BN) or Purging Disorder (PD)

Problem (P)	Etiology (E) (choose one)	Signs/Symptoms (S) (choose one or more)
Inadequate carbohydrate intake	Disordered eating Diagnosis of BN Harmful beliefs about eating	Avoidance of high-carbohydrate foods Irrational beliefs about the effects of carbohydrates on the body Insufficient intake of carbohydrate compared with estimated needs Hypoglycemia
Inadequate fluid intake	Excessive physical activity Disordered eating Harmful beliefs about drinking fluids	Acute weight loss Insufficient intake of fluids compared with estimated needs Elevated blood urea nitrogen (BUN) level Elevated sodium (Na) level Plasma or serum osmolality > 290 mOsm/kg
Harmful beliefs/attitudes about food and nutrition	Diagnosis of BN or PD Exposure to incorrect food and nutrition information	Intake reflecting an imbalance of food groups Irrational beliefs about the effects of food on the body Avoidance of food or food groups (specify) Food rituals (specify)

Continued on next page.

Table 3.2 (cont.) Sample Nutrition Diagnoses for Bulimia Nervosa (BN) or Purging Disorder (PD)

Problem (P)	Etiology (E) (choose one)	Signs/Symptoms (S) (choose one or more)
Disordered eating pattern	Obsessive desire to lose weight Undue influence of weight on self-esteem Diagnosis of BN	Abnormal laboratory values (specify) Purging Intake reflecting an imbalance of food groups Irrational beliefs about the effects of food on the body Avoidance of food or food groups (specify) Food rituals (specify)
Excessive exercise	Obsessive desire to lose weight Harmful beliefs about food	Irrational beliefs about the effects of food on the body Exercising when sick, injured or in defiance of medical recommendations Neglect of family, work or other responsibilities to exercise Exercise exceeding levels needed to improve health or athletic performance

Table 3.3 Sample Nutrition Diagnoses for Binge Eating Disorder and Night Eating Syndrome

Problem (P)	Etiology (E) (choose one)	Signs/Symptoms (S) (choose one or more)
Excessive energy intake Excessive oral food/ beverage intake	Disordered eating Diagnosis of binge eating disorder (BED) or night eating syndrome (NES)	Body fat > 32% (women) or > 25% (men) BMI > 25 (adults) or > 95th percentile Weight gain Intake of high caloric density or large portions of food/ beverages Binge eating Eating a majority of total caloric intake during the nighttime hours
Excessive fluid intake	Disordered eating Diagnosis of BED or NES Harmful beliefs about eating	Water or noncaloric beverage intake exceeding estimated needs Hyponatremia
Disordered eating pattern	Obsessive desire to lose weight Undue influence of weight on self-esteem Diagnosis of BED or NES	Restriction of food leading to binge eating Emotional eating Intake reflecting an imbalance of food groups

Continued on next page.

Table 3.3 (cont.) Sample Nutrition Diagnoses for Binge Eating Disorder (BED) and Night Eating Syndrome (NES)

Problem (P)	Etiology (E) (choose one)	Signs/Symptoms (S) (choose one or more)
Excessive exercise	Obsessive desire to lose weight Diagnosis of BED or NES Harmful beliefs about food	Irrational beliefs about the effects of food on the body Exercising when sick, injured, or in defiance of medical recommendations Neglect of family, work, or other responsibilities to exercise Exercise exceeding levels needed to improve health or athletic performance
Overweight/ obesity	Disordered eating pattern Diagnosis of BED or NES Excess energy intake Excess fluid intake Psychological stress History of abuse regarding weight or eating	BMI > 25 (overweight) or BMI > 30 (obesity) (adult) Weight for height above normative standard for age and gender (child) Increased body adiposity Increased skinfold thickness Overconsumption of calorie dense food/ beverages or large portions Binge eating Emotional eating

Chapter 4

Nutrition Intervention for Eating Disorders: Food and/or Nutrient Delivery and Nutrition-Related Medications

Based on your nutrition assessment and input from other providers working with each patient, you and the treatment team will plan how to proceed with a nutrition intervention.[1] Nutrition interventions for individuals with eating disorders will likely touch on all four categories in the Nutrition Care Process: Food and/or Nutrient Delivery, Nutrition Education, Nutrition Counseling, and Coordination of Nutrition Care.

Although nutrition diagnoses will vary from patient to patient, the goals of nutrition interventions tend to be very similar, even for different diagnoses. This is because consistent, basic, nutritious, balanced, varied, moderate eating is the foundation for recovery from all eating disorders.[1-7] General parameters for eating disorder recovery are summarized in Box 4.1 (see page 86).

The registered dietitian nutritionist (RDN) plays a role in each of these goal areas, with the greatest impact in the areas of improved nutrition status and "normalized" eating. For most patients, you will identify more than one nutrition intervention as necessary for the patient's health and nutritional restoration. Your primary challenge will be prioritizing interventions when many modifications are needed. Because a patient's ability to participate in eating disorder recovery depends on adequate nourishment to support cohesive thought, nutritional stability is a priority above all else except for physical safety and medical stability.[5]

Box 4.1 Indicators of Recovery from Eating Disorders

Ultimate treatment goals for all eating disorder types include:

- Medical and physical stability and physical health restoration
- "Normalized" (nonrestrictive) eating, including variety, balance, and nutritional adequacy without rigid guidelines for when, how, and why to eat or avoid certain foods
- "Normalized" physical activity, (not excessive, compulsive, or avoided) not used as a purging method or when injured and with adequate nutritional intake to fuel physical activities
- Absence of purging behaviors
- Healthy "coping mechanisms" (ways of dealing with stress) for stressors that formerly triggered eating disorder behaviors
- Improved mental health
- Supportive social structure in place to prevent relapse during stress

Meals and Snacks

The control of Food and/or Nutrient Delivery spans a continuum from the highest to the lowest levels of care.[1] An individual's ability or inability to meet his or her nutrition needs is in fact one of the major factors in determining which level of care is appropriate. In the higher levels of care (inpatient, residential, day treatment), the patient may have little or no control over food choices or method of delivery, leaving the RDN with full responsibility for diet orders and menus.[5] In the lower levels of care (intensive outpatient, outpatient), the RDN is limited to offering advice about food, and the patient bears all responsibility for obtaining, preparing, and consuming it. As patients transition through the levels, often RDNs and patients share these responsibilities.

As with all nutrition interventions, dietary recommendations will vary with each individual's nutrition assessment, diagnosis, and specific concerns. Because the long-term goal for nearly all patients with eating disorders is to achieve a more normalized and self-directed eating pattern, general guidelines can be applied, at least initially, in many cases. Table 4.1 lists sample nutrition interventions for each eating disorder diagnosis (see pages 88–92). You may pick and choose which interventions fit each individual's needs.

You will notice that there is no standard Food and/ or Nutrient Delivery Intervention specified for *type* of meal-planning method. This is because there is no one best way to structure a meal plan.[4] Your criteria for choosing a meal-planning method will not depend on an individual's diagnosis but rather on your facility's protocol (if applicable) blended with your patient's learning style, preferences, and need for structure.

If a patient has previously used a certain type of meal plan with success, you may consider using it as written, if appropriate, or adapting that structure to the patient's current needs. In cases where a patient used a past meal plan in a destructive manner, you may "start from scratch." Options for meal planning are summarized in Box 4.2.

Box 4.2 Meal-Planning Methods

- Fully prepared meals (eg, from an outside delivery service, a caregiver, or your facility's kitchen) based on your meal pattern and dietary recommendations

- Daily menus (RDN or patient with supervision of RDN writes out exactly what will be served at each meal or snack time)

- Meal schedule only (RDN or patient with RDN supervision plans meal and snack times; patient chooses from available foods at each time)

- Daily food group goals (a certain number of foods from each group eaten each day, but no specific goals as to which foods are eaten at which times)

- Exchange lists[8]

- Calorie counting (Because of the obsessive nature of eating disorders, use caution when choosing calorie counting as a teaching tool. Although it is of course appropriate for the RDN and hospital staff to document calories eaten in the medical record, dietitians are not encouraged to teach

Continued on next page.

Box 4.2 Meal-Planning Methods

calorie counting to patients with eating disorders in situations where the patient is likely to use calorie counting in a destructive or restrictive manner. If a patient is already counting calories as part of his or her eating disorder, an individual decision should be made by the RDN, patient, and treatment team whether to teach the patient a different meal-planning technique or whether to instead make use of the patient's existing knowledge of calorie counting to support a more appropriate calorie level.)

- Create Your Plate ("The Plate Method")[9]
- Others developed by individual dietitians, authors, and facilities

Meal Planning and Intuitive Eating

If you are familiar with nondiet, Health At Every Size, or intuitive eating philosophies, you may worry that meal planning for an individual with an eating disorder is the equivalent of "putting them on a diet." Because calorie-restricted diets are the trigger for many an eating disorder, you are wise to avoid encouraging further dieting behavior.[10,11] However, a meal plan devised by you should not be considered the equivalent of a diet, as it has five essential differences, as summarized in Box 4.3 on page 93.

Although your ultimate goal is for your patient to be able to eat intuitively, that is, based on internal cues, personal taste preferences, and changing individual needs, in most cases this cannot be your initial nutrition intervention. The vast majority of patients in your care for treatment of an eating disorder need some kind of structure from you in order to relearn appropriate hunger cues.[3,5]

Even if an individual initially expresses a desire to follow internal cues rather than a meal plan, it is not likely that he or she has the normal cues and responses that would be

Food or Nutrient Intervention	Anorexia Nervosa or Avoidant Restrictive Food Intake Disorder	Bulimia or Purging Disorder	Binge Eating Disorder or Night Eating Syndrome
Meals	3 per day	3 per day	3 per day
Snacks	3 or more per day as needed to provide adequate calories	0–3 per day as needed to maintain stable blood glucose levels depending on time period between meals	0–3 per day as needed to maintain stable blood glucose levels depending on time period between meals
Meal or snack timing	Evenly spaced, based on work or school schedule if appropriate. Times should be determined in advance and maintained as much as possible day to day	Based on patient preferences and work or school schedule if appropriate. Times should be determined in advance and maintained as much as possible day to day	Based on patient preferences and work or school schedule if appropriate. Times should be determined in advance and maintained as much as possible day to day
Meal or snack spacing	As needed to provide adequate intake	Avoid lengthy periods (>4–5 h) between meals or snacks	Avoid lengthy periods (>4–5 h) between meals or snacks
Meal or snack size and volume	Small portions to start, then advance as tolerated to meet energy needs	Small portions to start, then advance as tolerated to meet energy needs without purging	Modify as appropriate to meet energy needs

Table 4.1 Nutrition Intervention Guidelines for Eating Disorders: Meals and Snacks

Continued on next page.

Table 4.1 (cont.) Nutrition Intervention Guidelines for Eating Disorders: Meals and Snacks			
Food or Nutrient Intervention	Anorexia Nervosa or Avoidant Restrictive Food Intake Disorder	Bulimia or Purging Disorder	Binge Eating Disorder or Night Eating Syndrome
Meal or snack content	Estimate current daily intake, increase by 100–200 calories per day (inpatient) or 100–200 calories per week (outpatient) until meeting weight goals. Use preferences to start, advance to meet macronutrient needs, then incorporate balance and variety as tolerated. Limit noncaloric condiments and nonnutritive sweeteners. Do not provide foods known to cause purging or other self-harming behaviors unless supervision is provided	Include protein, carbohydrate, and fat sources at each meal, per patient preferences to start, advance to meet macronutrient needs, then incorporate balance and variety as tolerated. Limit noncaloric condiments and nonnutritive sweeteners. Avoid foods known to cause reflux or indigestion. Do not include foods known to cause bingeing or purging or other self-harming behaviors unless supervision is provided	Include protein, carbohydrate, and fat sources at each meal, follow patient preferences as possible, then incorporate balance and variety as tolerated. Do not include foods known to be triggers for bingeing or other self-harming behaviors unless supervision is provided

Continued on next page.

Table 4.1 (cont.) Nutrition Intervention Guidelines for Eating Disorders: Meals and Snacks			
Food or Nutrient Intervention	Anorexia Nervosa or Avoidant Restrictive Food Intake Disorder	Bulimia or Purging Disorder	Binge Eating Disorder or Night Eating Syndrome
Meal or snack duration	May require time limits to prevent prolonged meals, eg, 10–15 min per snack, 20–40 min per meal	May benefit from recommended meal duration to promote slow or appropriate pace of eating or pause partway through meal for 3–5 min	May benefit from recommended meal duration to promote slow or appropriate pace of eating or pause partway through meal for 3–5 min
Meal or snack supervision	May require supervision to discourage hiding, concealing, or destroying food. May benefit from support after eating to process feelings of distress and to discourage purging or other self-harming behaviors	May require supervision to discourage purging or other self-harming behaviors after eating. May require supervision using the bathroom. May benefit from support after meals to process feelings of distress. If meal preparation or cleanup trigger bingeing, delegate these tasks to others or provide supervision	As needed. May benefit from supervision or eating meals with others to encourage slow pace of eating, decrease of shame-based eating behavior, and social interaction. If meal preparation or cleanup trigger bingeing, delegate these tasks to others or provide supervision

Continued on next page.

Table 4.1 (cont.) Nutrition Intervention Guidelines for Eating Disorders: Meals and Snacks			
Food or Nutrient Intervention	Anorexia Nervosa or Avoidant Restrictive Food Intake Disorder	Bulimia or Purging Disorder	Binge Eating Disorder or Night Eating Syndrome
Meal or snack behavior	Discourage food rituals. Conversation should not focus on food	Discourage food rituals. Conversation should not focus on food. Address mindful eating and stress management before and after eating	Discourage food rituals. Conversation should not focus on food. Address mindful eating and stress management before eating
Meal or snack documentation	Document intake, have caregiver record initially if veracity is questionable. Specify if you prefer a percentage of meal consumed or specific foods	Document intake, bingeing, or bingeing triggers. Specify level of detail and which details are helpful. Document any compensatory behaviors	Document intake, bingeing, or bingeing triggers. Specify level of detail and which details are helpful

Continued on next page.

Table 4.1 (cont.) Nutrition Intervention Guidelines for Eating Disorders: Meals and Snacks

Food or Nutrient Intervention	Anorexia Nervosa or Avoidant Restrictive Food Intake Disorder	Bulimia or Purging Disorder	Binge Eating Disorder or Night Eating Syndrome
Beverage intake	If difficulty tolerating volume, limit beverages during meals to 8 oz. Limit caffeinated or non-caloric beverages. If patient complains of excessive thirst, evaluate medications and discuss with physician. If patient is dependent on caffeine, discuss weaning program with treatment team	If difficulty tolerating volume, limit beverages at mealtimes to 8 oz. Limit caffeinated or non-caloric beverages. Carbonated beverages can be used to help induce vomiting; limit as needed. If patient complains of excessive thirst, evaluate medications and discuss with physician. If patient is dependent on caffeine, discuss weaning program with treatment team	Limit caloric beverages as needed. If patient complains of excessive thirst, evaluate medications and discuss with physician. If patient is dependent on caffeine, discuss weaning program with treatment team

Box 4.3 How Your Meal Plan Is Unlike a Diet

Your meal plan is devised to promote physical and mental health for your patient, not to destroy health in search of weight loss at any cost.

Your meal plan is (ultimately) intended to provide *adequate* calories, rather than calorie deprivation, which is the goal of all weight-loss diets. Adequate caloric intake, even if it is fewer total calories than the patient's current intake, as in the case of binge eating disorder, will not trigger the starvation mechanisms and eating-disordered responses that weight-loss diets cause.

Your meal plan is individualized to each patient. Even though you may use your facility's general protocol as a starting point, unlike weight-loss diets that are standard for everyone, your meal plan will ultimately be unique for each and every patient.

Your meal plan is modifiable, with input from the patient. Unlike rigid weight-loss diets that require the dieter to meet the same calorie goals with the same allowed foods and the same disallowed foods week after week after week, your meal plan will be adapted by you and your patient on a daily, weekly, or other basis, based on the patient's changing (and hopefully improving) sense of taste, satiety, activity level, and other needs and desires.

Someday your meal plan will be obsolete. It is simply a tool to teach patients to nourish themselves without the need of a meal plan at all. This is the polar opposite of weight-loss diets that tout themselves as "a lifestyle" that requires constant participation and purchases.

---

required to do so.[1] Long-held habits and food rules are difficult to break, even when you give a patient good information. It is difficult to connect with internal cues after months or years of ignoring hunger by restricting or pushing past fullness when binge eating. Anxiety about food and the stress hormones it triggers interfere with the ability to sense hunger and fullness. Early satiety, delayed gastric emptying, bloating or nausea may be misinterpreted as "fullness" and therefore a reason to stop eating too early or to purge.[3]

The occasional exception is the highly functioning individual who comes to you in the outpatient setting self-diagnosed with "an eating disorder." This type of patient would be more appropriately categorized as a "disordered eater" confused about what, when, and why to eat, with dieting rules that lead to occasional binge eating. The patient may be able to eat intuitively but has not been exposed to the idea. He or she may fear that intuitive eating would cause weight gain but is willing to trial it under your supervision. This type of patient would benefit from your guidance in attending to hunger and satiety cues, and your education that intuitive eating is more likely to lead to a "natural" weight than to weight gain specifically. "Disordered eating" may respond very well to the teachings of intuitive eating, but an individual with a true eating disorder will need to learn intuitive eating principles further into recovery, after the initial principles of good nutrition have been met and the patient is physically and mentally stable.[3]

For patients who continue to meet with you over time, your role will change as recovery progresses.[4] Assistance in identifying hunger cues *while still following the meal plan* is a next step and should be practiced under your supervision before an individual attempts to eat solely in response to hunger cues.[3] A severely ill patient in the initial stages of treatment may express a desire to control his or her meal plan and may resist allowing you to take the lead. However, the patient, at this point, is not likely to benefit from providing input into the meal plan; you should take on this role at first.

A medically well outpatient, conversely, might need very little guidance from you on exactly what to eat but more education in portion sizes, observing hunger cues, and other nutrition topics covered in "Nutrition Education" (see Chapter 5). And when individuals who are mapping their own meal plans need to plan ahead for a new or stressful eating situation, they may benefit from more hands-on advice from you than in a more typical or ordinary situation.

Your flexibility to offer more or less structure without judgment is a strength that will support your patient in feeling safe to ask for help when needed.[4,12,13] Many patients are eventually able to manage their own meal schedule and decision making, maintaining an appropriate body weight using their internal cues as a guide. At this time we are unable to predict how long each individual must wait for his or her hunger patterns to return. Research on appetite-related hormones, such as leptin, ghrelin, cholecystokinin, adiponectin, insulin, and others, may add to our knowledge in this area.[14-16]

Medical Food Supplements

The need and desire to use meal replacement beverages, supplemental oral nutritional formulas, and other medical food supplements (puddings, shakes, and so forth) will differ from patient to patient. Some individuals with eating disorders prefer food: Their point of view is, "If I have to get the calories, I want to enjoy them." Others fear that if they eat and enjoy food, they will become overeaters. They prefer to ingest additional calories via supplements that seem more like medicine than food. Individuals experiencing depression and its associated lack of interest in food may simply not have the motivation or desire to purchase, prepare, or even consume regular food.[17] Still others enjoy their nutrition supplements or enjoy their abnormality; they are not willing to give up the perceived cachet of having an eating disorder yet.

Regardless of the patient's motive, supplemental nutrition is a useful tool to increase caloric intake beyond what the patient is willing or able to eat from food.[5,18] Additionally, it provides a balance of nutrients in situations where oral food intake is unbalanced or rigid. Many individuals receiving treatment for anorexia require far more calories than expected in order to gain weight.[19-21] In these cases of hypermetabolism, where the energy cost of weight restoration is far higher than eventual (normalized) energy needs, supplementation with a high-calorie liquid supplement can be a welcome relief. This offers the patient the opportunity to learn and practice eating a "normal" volume of food, while supplementing to meet additional calorie needs. Once metabolism has normalized, the patient can simply discontinue the supplementation while keeping food intake stable.

Philosophies differ among experts as to how long a person should be encouraged to use supplemental nutrition rather than meeting needs from food. Some patients will need encouragement to transition from supplements to food; others will wean themselves naturally as their recovery progresses. Others may continue to supplement because of convenience, preference, or habit long after their other eating behaviors have normalized. This is a decision that you and your treatment team should make, usually together with each patient, on a case-by-case basis.

Enteral and Parenteral Nutrition

Enteral nutrition ("tube feeding") is an option for individuals with eating disorders who are unable or unwilling to meet their energy needs with food or oral supplementation.[18-25] If a patient is in this situation, the treatment team should discuss the pros and cons with the patient; knowing that tube feeding is imminent occasionally motivates patients to meet their needs by mouth. Using enteral nutrition as a threat, however, is not recommended,[6] nor is excessive attention, which can reward and reinforce aspects of the eating disorder.[23] As a medical procedure, it should be initiated when medically necessary and appropriate.

Total parenteral nutrition (TPN) and peripheral parenteral nutrition (PPN) are rarely initiated for individuals with eating disorders, as neither encourages the healthy eating behaviors and hunger cues necessary for recovery.[5,22] TPN should be used only when absolutely necessary and for the shortest possible duration. Examples include a patient with an eating disorder who also has pancreatitis; a patient whose energy needs for weight restoration are so exorbitant that they cannot be met by a combination of oral and enteral feeding; or a patient who disconnects, contaminates, refuses, or purges enteral feedings even when supervised. Box 4.4 summarizes possible indications for enteral and parenteral feedings for eating disorders.

Family members may have strong feelings or misconceptions regarding nutrition support and, if so, will need education and guidance in response to their concerns.

Refeeding Syndrome

Any starved patient who begins the process of nutritional rehabilitation can experience symptoms as the body readjusts from the malnourished, metabolic conservation mode into a more normal utilization of energy and nutrients.[18-25] This includes individuals with eating disorders who have experienced self-imposed starvation or consumed extremely limited calories for a period of time. These symptoms may be uncomfortable and annoying, such as flatulence, constipation, nausea, diarrhea, and bloating, or they may be dangerous and life-threatening, such as electrolyte imbalance and heart failure. The most severe of these symptoms are called "refeeding syndrome" and can be fatal, however, with appropriate monitoring, risk can be greatly reduced.[24-29]

Refeeding syndrome occurs when adaptations to starvation are rapidly reversed. Laboratory values that appear normal or near normal in the initial malnourished state (because of adaptations to starvation and dehydration) mask the true medical frailty of the patient. When enteral or aggressive oral feeding begin, these laboratory values may suddenly decrease. Careful, daily monitoring of

**Box 4.4 Sample Enteral and Parenteral Nutrition
Interventions for Eating Disorders[a,5,6,22]**

Sample Situation	Possible Intervention
At each meal, the patient is offered a tray. Each time, the patient refuses any oral caloric intake.	Initiate nasogastric (NG) tube feeding and increase as tolerated. Each time the patient refuses oral intake, provide a bolus feeding of equivalent calories. Hold tube feeding if the patient is willing to eat a full meal. Discontinue tube feeding when the patient is willing and able to meet 90%–100% of nutrition needs by mouth (PO) (all meals and snacks) for 48 hours.
At each meal, the patient eats some food but refuses to finish the meal. Patient is offered an oral nutrition supplement equal to uneaten calories but refuses.	Initiate NG tube feeding and increase as tolerated. Each time the patient refuses to finish the meal, estimate the remaining (uneaten) calories and provide a bolus feeding of equivalent calories. Hold tube feeding if the patient is willing to eat a full meal. Discontinue tube feeding when the patient is willing and able to meet 90%–100% of nutrition needs PO (all meals and snacks) for 48 hours.
The patient is eating, but due to poor appetite or fear of weight gain, is not able to eat enough to prevent additional weight loss.	Initiate NG tube feeding and increase as tolerated. Allow the patient to eat according to the meal plan during the day. Subtract calories eaten from the total needs; provide necessary additional calories continuously through the night until 3–4 hours before breakfast to promote a normal pattern of hunger. Discontinue tube feeding when the patient is able to meet 90%–100% of nutrition needs PO.

Continued on next page.

Box 4.4 (cont.) Sample Enteral and Parenteral Nutrition Interventions for Eating Disorders[a,5,6,22]

Sample Situation	Possible Intervention
The patient is unable to think clearly, make competent decisions, or proceed in treatment due to malnutrition.	Initiate NG tube feeding and provide total calories over a 24-hour continuous drip. Once 100% of nutrient needs are being met, advance as tolerated to bolus feedings at meal and snack times to promote a normal pattern of hunger. Once the patient begins eating, subtract calories eaten from the tube feeding. Transition to nighttime tube feeding if patient is able to eat during the day. Discontinue tube feeding when the patient is able to meet 90%–100% of nutrition needs PO.
The patient is eating but is unable to meet the excessive energy needs of hypermetabolism.	Initiate NG tube feeding and increase as tolerated. Allow the patient to eat as possible throughout the day. Subtract calories eaten from total needs; provide necessary additional calories continuously through the night until 3–4 hours before breakfast to promote a normal pattern of hunger. Discontinue tube feeding when the metabolic rate normalizes and the patient is able to meet 90%–100% of nutrient needs PO.
The patient is medically unstable and, although willing to eat, is not able to meet nutrition needs with food.	Initiate NG tube feeding and provide total calories over a 24-hour continuous drip. Allow the patient to eat as possible during the day, but do not subtract from the tube feeding. Once 100% of the nutrient needs are being met via tube feeding, subtract the eaten calories from the tube feeding total. Continue to decrease tube feeding as PO intake increases. Discontinue tube feeding once the patient is medically stable or able to meet 90%–100% nutrient needs PO.

Continued on next page.

**Box 4.4 (cont.) Sample Enteral and Parenteral Nutrition
Interventions for Eating Disorders**[a,5,6,22]

Sample Situation	Possible Intervention
The patient has gastrointestinal (GI) dysfunction, such as involuntary regurgitation of food (gut rest not required).	Initiate NG or nasojejunal (NJ) tube feeding, depending on the location of the GI dysfunction, and advance as tolerated to provide total calories over a 24-hour continuous drip. Once GI function is restored, allow the patient to trial a full liquid diet, then progress as tolerated to small, easily digestible foods while providing additional needed calories via tube feeding. Discontinue tube feeding when the patient is able to meet and keep down 90%–100% of nutrition needs PO.
The patient has not met a goal weight or intake level previously agreed on by the treatment team.	Initiate tube feeding and advance as tolerated. Tube feed according to agreed-on plan.
The patient is unable to meet energy needs via a combination of oral and enteral feeding.	Supplemental PPN
The patient requires total gut rest or cannot tolerate enteral feeding due to pancreatitis, GI blockage, or other medical condition.	TPN
The patient sabotages or refuses oral and enteral feeding even when supervised.	TPN

[a] Note: Nutrition support is not a punishment and should not be referred to as such.

phosphorous, potassium, magnesium, calcium, and sodium levels together with slow increases in tube-feeding volume provide the best defense against such complications, especially during the first week of nutritional rehabilitation. Individuals most at risk are those who weigh less than 70% of usual or expected body weight or have lost more than 10% of their body weight in the past 3 months.[24]

Box 4.5 provides guidelines for initiating and advancing enteral feeding in a malnourished patient in order to best decrease the risk of refeeding syndrome.[29] At times it may seem counterproductive to advance enteral nutrition at a slower than desired pace, but prevention of refeeding syndrome takes priority. Work closely with your patient's medical team to determine when it is appropriate to advance tube-feeding rate, volume, and caloric density.

Vitamin and Mineral Supplements

It is common sense that an individual with difficulty eating is likely to have nutritional deficiencies; however, there is no way to predict micronutrient deficiencies by diagnosis alone. Because each person with an eating disorder has his or her own combination of eating practices, resulting in potential deficiencies and excessive intakes of different micronutrients, each patient must be evaluated individually by an RDN. During this process, you will observe a variety of combinations of included and excluded foods and food groups, which will provide you clues to the most likely micronutrient deficiencies. Some individuals attempt to avoid all foods containing more than trace amounts of dietary fat, resulting in inadequate absorption of fat-soluble nutrients. Others restrict meats and dairy products without substituting suitable vegetarian alternatives, leading to deficiencies in nutrients primarily found in animal foods. In other cases, patients ingest excessive quantities of certain items or eat the same few nutritionally limited foods over

---

Box 4.5 Guidelines for Enteral Feeding to Decrease Risk of Refeeding Syndrome[5,6,22]

Protein repletion should begin at 1.2–1.5 g protein per kg ideal body weight in order to protect lean body tissue despite a hypo-caloric diet.

Initially, calories should be in accordance with intake during starvation, and the infusion should not exceed 25–50 cc/h from the tube. Rapid progression increases the likelihood of complications. Maintain the patient on a hypocaloric diet through the first 3–5 days. Then gradually adjust calories upward toward the full needs as tolerated. This may mean daily adjustments as minimal as 0–150 kcal per day until you are certain tolerance is consistent.

An isotonic, fiber-containing, polymeric formula is usually sufficient for nutritional repletion, unless impaired digestion or absorption indicates use of an elemental diet, medium-chain triglyceride (MCT) oil, or peptide-based product. Maximize fat calories and avoid high-glucose formulas.

Fluid intolerance is exacerbated by excess carbohydrate introduction. At initiation of fluids, limit carbohydrate calories to 150–200 g/day at appropriately spaced intervals. Monitor carbohydrates in the meal plan and the feeding formula until weight gain is proven to be gradual and appropriate.

Recommended fluid intake for the low-weight individual is 20–50 cc water per kg body weight or 1 cc water per kcal formula.

Gradually increase the feedings by 10–25 cc/h every 8 to 24 hours if tolerated until the target rate is achieved. Weaning can begin as soon as the tube-feeding objectives are being met and medical complications are resolved.

Evaluate daily during the first week of enteral feeding: body weight and blood glucose, fluid input and output, serum electrolyte, blood urea nitrogen (BUN), and creatinine levels.

Evaluate weekly as enteral feeding continues: prealbumin, calcium, magnesium, phosphorus, potassium, sodium, BUN, and creatinine levels until stable.

---

and over again, resulting in extremely low intake of particular micronutrients.

Box 4.6 summarizes which micronutrients may be deficient in patients who have eliminated most or all foods in a certain food group.

Box 4.6 Potential Micronutrient Deficiencies Caused by Food Group Restriction	
Restricted or Eliminated Food Group	Micronutrients Potentially Deficient
Dairy products	Calcium, vitamin D, vitamin B-12
Vegetables	Fiber, potassium, folic acid, vitamin C
Meat, poultry, fish, eggs	Iron, zinc, selenium, magnesium, copper, vitamin B-12, omega-3 fatty acids
Fats, oils	Vitamin E; vitamins A and D, omega-3 fatty acids
Grains (bread, cereal, rice, pasta)	B vitamins
Fruits	Vitamins A and C, folic acid, potassium

Because nutritional issues vary from patient to patient, no standard recommendation exists for vitamin and mineral supplementation in eating disorders.[4,30] Studies attempting to determine the prevalence of micronutrient deficiencies in patients with eating disorders show conflicting results, likely caused by the frequent use of self-prescribed supplements and excessive use of hyperfortified processed foods. Clinical trials of individual micronutrient supplementation for purposes of improving depression or other symptoms of eating disorders or mental illness are appearing in the literature, but no consensus has been reached. It cannot be overstated, however, that simply reversing nutrient deficiencies is not the same as curing an eating disorder.

Even with your patient's own micronutrient laboratory test results in hand, a thorough dietary history is likely to paint a more accurate picture of potential nutrient deficiencies. Use your clinical judgment along with your assessment of eating behaviors to determine which micronutrients require supplementation.

Table 4.2 summarizes the available data on single-nutrient supplementation for individuals with eating disorders. Some treatment centers administer a daily multivitamin–mineral supplement to all patients admitted with eating disorders.[4] This is an acceptable baseline to which additional single-nutrient supplements can be added on an individual basis.

Table 4.2 Micronutrient Deficiencies and Supplementation Guidelines for Eating Disorders[30]

Nutrient	Preferred Method to Assess Deficiency in Eating Disordered Patients	Eating Disorder-Specific Supplementation Guidelines
Calcium[a]	Long-term: poor bone density Short-term: dietary inadequacy	Supplement with calcium citrate to total 1,500 mg/day elemental calcium from food and supplement. Divide calcium dose into 500 mg increments
Iron	Plasma ferritin < 30 ng/mL for men and < 15 ng/mL for women	Refer to physician for prescription. Long-term administration and monitoring necessary
Phosphate[a]	< 2.5 mg/dL	IV administration per patient needs
Potassium[a]	< 3.5 mEq/L	IV administration per patient needs
Magnesium[a]	< 1.5 mEq/L	IV administration per patient needs

Continued on next page.

Table 4.2 (cont.) Micronutrient Deficiencies and Supplementation Guidelines for Eating Disorders[30]

Nutrient	Preferred Method to Assess Deficiency in Eating Disordered Patients	Eating Disorder-Specific Supplementation Guidelines
Sodium[a]	< 136 mEq/L	IV administration per patient needs
Vitamin A (retinol, carotene)	Dietary inadequacy	700 mcg retinol/day (Recommended Dietary Allowance [RDA] for females > 14 years old) 900 mcg retinol/day (RDA for males > 14 years old) Supplementation above the RDA not recommended
Vitamin B-1 (thiamin, thiamine)	Dietary inadequacy Alcohol dependence	1.4 mg/day (RDA)
Vitamin B-2 (riboflavin)	Long-term: activity coefficient of erythrocyte glutathione reductase > 1.4 Short-term: dietary inadequacy	1.3 mg/day (RDA for men) 1.1 mg/day (RDA for women)
Vitamin B-6 (pyridoxine)	Dietary inadequacy Alcohol dependence	1.3 mg/day
Vitamin B-9 (folic acid)	Plasma folate ≤ 3 ng/ML or red blood cell folate of ≤ 140 ng/mL or elevated plasma homocysteine level	400 mcg/day

Continued on next page.

Table 4.2 (cont.) Micronutrient Deficiencies and Supplementation Guidelines for Eating Disorders[30]

Nutrient	Preferred Method to Assess Deficiency in Eating Disordered Patients	Eating Disorder-Specific Supplementation Guidelines
Vitamin B-12 (cobalamin)	< 200 pg/mL or elevated plasma homocysteine level	1 mg intramuscular (IM) cyanocobalamin/month or 2 mg oral cyanocobalamin/day
Vitamin C	Long-term: 2-hour urinary excretion < 28 mg, 4 h after preload of ascorbic acid Short-term: dietary inadequacy	Up to 400 mg/day
Vitamin D	25-hydroxyvitamin D < 20 ng/mL	No consensus
Zinc	Serum zinc < 46 ng/dL Hypogeusia (diminished sense of taste)	100 mg/day zinc gluconate (providing 14 mg/day elemental zinc)

[a] Note that abnormal blood value levels of these nutrients reflect long-term or serious whole-body deficiency. These should be referred for medical evaluation and should be checked daily during the first week of nutritional rehabilitation as levels can decrease even with supplementation.

Adapted with permission from Setnick J. Micronutrient Deficiencies and Supplementation in Anorexia and Bulimia Nervosa: A Review of Literature. *Nutr Clin Practice.* 2010;25(2):137-142.

Nutrition-Related Medication Management

Individuals with eating disorders often benefit from psychoactive medication and in many cases require it to treat co-occurring conditions. It is crucial that a psychiatrist or psychiatric nurse practitioner experienced with eating

disorders is a part of the treatment team. To date, no medications have been approved specifically to treat anorexia
nervosa; only fluoxetine has been Food and Drug Administration (FDA) approved to treat bulimia;[31] lisdexamfetamine
has been FDA approved to treat moderate to severe binge
eating disorder.[32] Topiramate has been considered by the
FDA for treatment of binge eating disorder, but it has not
yet been FDA approved for this purpose.[33] Once a drug is
FDA approved, it may be prescribed for other "off-label"
uses, and many are used as treatments for eating disorders
and their underlying and co-occurring disorders. When
matched with appropriate medication(s) and dosage by a
skilled professional, eating and mental symptoms markedly
improve for many eating disorder patients.

A minority of individuals with eating disorders react
to medication with a total remission of symptoms, no
benefit at all, or serious side effects. Sometimes several
medications are trialed before the best match is determined.
Ideally, each patient works with a prescribing professional
experienced with eating disorders who can monitor positive
and negative effects and modify prescriptions as needed.
Table 4.3 (pages 109–115) summarizes the known potential
nutrition-related effects.

Nutrition-Related Side Effects and Medication Abuse

The RDN's role expands when a psychoactive medication
is prescribed.[34,35] Medication and nutrition influence each
other, and medication efficacy may be enhanced or reduced
depending on nutrition status. Not every person will experience every side effect; nevertheless it is helpful for the
RDN to be aware of the potential concerns and to counsel
the individual accordingly. In an outpatient setting especially, the RDN may have the most frequent contact with

Table 4.3 Psychoactive Mediations with Potential Nutritional Effects[5,6,31,33-36]

Medication (Brand Name)	FDA Approved for Treatment of	Potential Nutrition Effects
Alprazolam (Xanax)	Anxiety	Appetite and weight either way
Aripiprazole (Abilify)	Bipolar disorder Schizophrenia Depression	Nausea Constipation Hyperglycemia Weight gain Orthostatic hypotension
Amitriptyline (Elavil)	Anxiety Depression	Appetite and weight up Carb and sweets cravings Increased blood glucose levels High fiber intake may decrease drug efficacy Increased need for riboflavin
Amphetamine salts (Adderall)[a]	Attention-deficit disorder (ADD) Attention-deficit with hyperactivity disorder (ADHD)	Appetite and weight down (can be dramatic) Difficulty gaining weight
Bupropion (Wellbutrin)	Depression Smoking cessation	Appetite and weight down
Carbamazepine (Tegretol, Equetro)	Bipolar disorder	Appetite down

Continued on next page.

Table 4.3 (cont.) Psychoactive Mediations with Potential Nutritional Effects[5,6,31,33-36]

Medication (Brand Name)	FDA Approved for Treatment of	Potential Nutrition Effects
Chlorpromazine (Thorazine)	Schizophrenia Anxiety	Appetite and weight up Increased cholesterol levels Increased blood glucose levels Increased need for riboflavin Cardiac complications
Citalopram (Celexa)	Depression	Weight gain possible
Clonazepam (Klonopin)	Anxiety	Appetite down Thirst up Weight either way
Clozapine (Clozaril)	Schizophrenia Anxiety	Weight gain (can be extreme) Severe constipation Cardiac complications Increased blood glucose levels Increased cholesterol levels New-onset diabetes mellitus
Desipramine (Norpramin)	Anxiety Depression	Appetite and weight up Sweets cravings High-fiber diet may decrease drug efficacy Increased need for riboflavin Increased glucose levels

Continued on next page.

Table 4.3 (cont.) Psychoactive Mediations with Potential Nutritional Effects[5,6,31,33-36]

Medication (Brand Name)	FDA Approved for Treatment of	Potential Nutrition Effects
Dextroam-phetamine (Dexedrine)[a]	ADHD	Appetite and weight down Calcium or magnesium supplements may increase drug effect Vitamin C supplement or acidic foods may decrease drug absorption
Doxepin (Sin-equan, Adapin)	Anxiety Depression	Appetite and weight up Thirst up Sweets cravings High-fiber diet may decrease efficacy Increased blood glucose levels
Duloxetine (Cymbalta)	Depression	Can affect appetite and weight either way
Escitalopram (Lexapro)	Depression	Appetite and weight up Increased cholesterol levels
Fluoxetine (Prozac)	Anxiety Depression Bulimia	Appetite and weight up
Flurazepam (Dalmane)	Insomnia	Can affect appetite and weight either way
Fluvoxamine (Luvox)	Obsessive-compulsive disorder Bulimia Schizophrenia Panic disorder	Appetite and weight either way Increased cholesterol levels

Continued on next page.

Table 4.3 (cont.) Psychoactive Mediations with Potential Nutritional Effects[5,6,31,33-36]

Medication (Brand Name)	FDA Approved for Treatment of	Potential Nutrition Effects
Lithium (Eskalith, Lithotabs, Lithonate, Lithane)	Bipolar disorder	Weight and thirst up Appetite down Recommend noncaloric beverages and consistent sodium intake Limit xanthine (coffee, tea, cola) Increased serum electrolyte levels Bloating
Lisdexamfetamine (Vyvanse)[a]	ADD/ADHD Binge eating disorder	Appetite and weight down (can be dramatic) Nausea
Lurasidone (Latuda)	Bipolar disorder	Nausea
Methylphenidate (Ritalin)[a]	ADD/ADHD	Appetite and weight down (can be dramatic) Difficulty gaining weight
Nortriptyline (Pamelor)	Anxiety Depression	Appetite and weight up Carb and sweets cravings Increased blood glucose levels High fiber intake may decrease drug efficacy Increased need for riboflavin

Continued on next page.

Table 4.3 (cont.) Psychoactive Mediations with Potential Nutritional Effects[5,6,31,33-36]

Medication (Brand Name)	FDA Approved for Treatment of	Potential Nutrition Effects
Olanzapine (Zyprexa)	Schizophrenia Anxiety	Appetite and weight up (can be dramatic and can cause diabetes or ketosis) Increased cholesterol or triglyceride levels Cardiac complications
Paroxetine (Paxil)	Anxiety Depression	Appetite and weight up (can be dramatic)
Pemoline (Cylert)	ADD	Appetite down (can be dramatic) Weight loss or difficulty gaining weight
Phenelzine (Nardil)	Depression	Appetite and weight up Monoamine oxidase inhibitor (MAOI)— limit high tyramine foods
Phenytoin (Dilantin)	Antiseizure	Decreased folate, Phosphorus, cholesterol, calcium, vitamin D levels Increased blood glucose levels Increased metabolism of vitamins D and K Folic acid supplement >5 mg/wk lowers drug availability Antacids, enteral feedings, and calcium supplements should be separated from drug administration by at least 2 h

Continued on next page.

Table 4.3 (cont.) Psychoactive Mediations with Potential Nutritional Effects[5,6,31,33-36]

Medication (Brand Name)	FDA Approved for Treatment of	Potential Nutrition Effects
Quetiapine (Seroquel)	Bipolar disorder Schizophrenia	Weight up Constipation Increased glucose and cholesterol levels
Risperidone (Risperdal)	Schizophrenia Anxiety	Appetite and weight up Sodium, hemoglobin, hematocrit levels down Cardiac complications Increased glucose levels
Sertraline (Zoloft)	Anxiety Depression	Appetite and weight either way GI upset
Thioridazine (Mellaril)	Schizophrenia Anxiety	Appetite and weight up Increased cholesterol and glucose levels Increased need for riboflavin Cardiac complications
Thiothixene (Navane)	Schizophrenia Anxiety	Appetite and weight up Increased need for riboflavin Cardiac complications
Topiramate (Topamax)	Binge eating disorder	Decreased impulse to binge Decreased appetite Weight loss Increased lactic acid levels Metabolic acidosis Kidney stones
Trazodone (Desyrel)	Depression Insomnia	Appetite and weight either way Anemia Edema

Continued on next page.

Table 4.3 (cont.) Psychoactive Mediations with Potential Nutritional Effects[5,6,31,33-36]		
Medication (Brand Name)	**FDA Approved for Treatment of**	**Potential Nutrition Effects**
Valproic acid (Depakote)	Bipolar disorder	Appetite and weight increase
		Increased cholesterol levels
		False-positive ketones test results
		GI distress
		Polycystic ovary syndrome
		Altered thyroid function tests
Venlafaxine (Effexor)	Anxiety Depression Panic disorder	Appetite and weight either way
Zolpidem (Ambien)	Insomnia	Binge eating or night eating with amnesia, leading to weight gain

ªDue to their dramatic appetite-inhibiting side effects, these stimulant medications are vulnerable as drugs of abuse among patients with eating disorders.

the patient and may recognize medication side effects that patients are attributing to increased eating or to certain foods. Appropriately ascribing these side effects, such as GI distress, to medications rather than food can improve the patient's willingness to continue nutritional rehabilitation.[34]

Medications with appetite-inhibiting side effects provide the greatest challenge for individuals who need to increase their intake. Confer with the prescribing professional to determine if the timing of dosage can be moved from before eating to after eating or entirely separate from mealtime.

Patients who induce vomiting immediately or a short time after taking their medication may not receive the full effects of their medication. This should be addressed either via changing the timing of meals, the timing of medication (with supervision of the prescribing professional), or behavioral intervention.

Medications with weight gain side effects can be particularly distressing to individuals with eating disorders, regardless of their current weight. If a patient is at a healthy weight and gaining, overweight, or gaining weight rapidly without a concurrent change in eating, this is a side effect that needs to be reported to the prescribing professional. In some cases alternatives exist. When there is no other medication that can be used, support your patient in following his or her meal plan rather than returning to eating disorder behaviors.[30]

Certain medications are weight-dependent and may require adjustment of dosages with major changes in weight. Report large weight changes over time to the prescribing physician. With medications that increase thirst or cause a feeling of dryness in the mouth, unnecessary weight gain can be mediated by recommending that your patient reduce his or her intake of calorie-containing beverages.[36] Daily calorie intake may be dramatically reduced by a switch to water or other low-calorie beverages.

Encourage patients to report all side effects (nutrition-related and otherwise), especially increased thoughts of self-harm or suicide. Do not recommend that a patient discontinue a medication as some substances build up in the bloodstream over time and require a weaning protocol to avoid complications. If a patient reports noncompliance with medication to you (over- or under-dosing, or use other than as prescribed) or reveals that he or she has run out of a prescribed medication, you or the patient should report this right away to a member of the medical team who can advise the patient.

Some eating disorder patients abuse prescription or over-the-counter (OTC) preparations. This should be reported to the psychiatrist on the team, or a referral should be made if the patient has not had a psychiatric evaluation. Although inappropriate, this type of drug use may point to a legitimate need for medication. There is one important exception: If a patient is abusing ipecac syrup as a means to induce vomiting, he or she should be counseled to stop immediately, and the physician should be notified. Ipecac syrup builds up in the body and can be lethal.

Resistance to Medication

You may encounter reluctance from a patient or family members to consider using psychoactive medication, or even to simply meet with a psychiatrist. In these situations, it is important that your personal preferences and opinions regarding medication do not influence your professionalism. It is always appropriate to encourage the patient and family to bring any medication-related concerns directly to the physician, psychiatrist, nurse practitioner, nurse, or other member of the medical team who can provide more information about the rationale for and risks and benefits of medication.

Because eating disorder behaviors cause calming or "self-medicating" effects, a patient may describe feeling addicted to the behaviors or the relief that they temporarily provide.

Psychoactive medications, although not prescribed to counter a specific eating disorder behavior, can promote improved mental health, stop obsessive thoughts and ruminations, decrease paralyzing depression or anxiety, and allow for clearer thinking, therefore promoting eating disorder recovery.

Although it may seem to be a trial and error process, medications can be a hugely important and sometimes essential piece of the recovery puzzle. Once the eating disorder is in remission (generally defined as 6 months completely symptom free), individuals who would like to attempt recovery without medication can raise the issue with their physician. If the decision is made to decrease or discontinue a medication, all treatment team members including the patient should be alert for any flare up in symptoms or behaviors that may occur.

References

1. American Dietetic Association. Position of the American Dietetic Association: nutrition intervention in the treatment of eating disorders. *J Am Diet Assoc.* 2011;111(8):1236-1241.

2. Gilbert SD, Commerford MC. *The Unofficial Guide to Managing Eating Disorders.* Foster City, VA: IDG Books Worldwide; 2000.

3. Tribole E. Intuitive eating in the treatment of eating disorders: the journey of attunement. *Renfrew Perspect.* 2010;(Winter):11-14.

4. Reiter CS, Graves L. Nutrition therapy for eating disorders. *Nutr Clin Pract.* 2010;25:122-136.

5. Yager J, Devlin MJ, Halmi KA, et al. *Practice Guideline for the Treatment of Patients with Eating Disorders.* 3rd ed. Arlington, VA: American Psychiatric Association; 2006.

6. Setnick J. *The Eating Disorders Clinical Pocket Guide: Quick Reference for Healthcare Providers.* Dallas, TX: Snack Time Press; 2005.

7. Kratina K. Health at every size: clinical applications. *Healthy Weight J.* 2003;17(2):19-23.

8. American Dietetic Association and American Diabetes Association. *Choose Your Foods: Exchange Lists for Diabetes.* Chicago, IL: American Dietetic Association; 2008.

9. American Diabetes Association. Create your plate.
    www.diabetes.org/food-and-fitness/food/plan-
    ning-meals/create-your-plate/. Accessed August 20,
    2010.

10. Tribole E, Resch E. *Intuitive Eating: A Revolutionary
    Program That Works.* 2nd ed. New York: St. Martin's
    Griffin; 2003.

11. Vredrvelt P, Newman D, Beverly H, Minirth F. *The
    Thin Disguise: Understanding and Overcoming
    Anorexia and Bulimia.* Nashville, TN: Thomas Nel-
    son; 1992.

12. Kellogg M. *Counseling Tips for Nutrition Thera-
    pists: Practice Workbook.* Vol 1. Philadelphia, PA: Kg
    Press; 2006.

13. Kellogg M. *Counseling Tips for Nutrition Thera-
    pists: Practice Workbook.* Vol 2. Philadelphia, PA: Kg
    Press; 2009.

14. Esterling E, Neubauer S. The relationship of ghrelin
    to appetite and weight management. *Weight Manage
    Matters.* 2008;6(2):1-24.

15. Thomas S, Schauer P. Bariatric surgery and the gut
    hormone response. *Nutr Clin Pract.* 2010;25:175-182.

16. Bacon L. Tales of mice and leptin: false promises
    and new hope in weight control. *Healthy Weight J.*
    2003;17(2):24-27.

17. American Psychiatric Association. *The Diagnostic
    and Statistical Manual of Mental Disorders.* 5th ed.
    Arlington, VA: American Psychiatric Association;
    2013.

18. Tresley J, Sheean PM. Refeeding syndrome: recogni-
    tion is the key to prevention and management. *J Am
    Diet Assoc.* 2008;108: 2105-2108.

19. Moukaddem M, Bouier A, Apfelbaum M, Rigaud D.
    Increase in diet-induced thermogenesis at the start of
    refeeding in severely malnourished anorexia nervosa
    patients. *Am Soc Clin Nutr.* 1997;66:133-140.

20. Schebendach JE, Golden NH, Jacobson MS, Hertz S, Shenker IR. The metabolic responses to starvation and refeeding in adolescents with anorexia nervosa. *Ann N Y Acad Sci.* 1997;817:110-119.

21. Salisbury JJ, Levine AS, Crow SJ, Mitchell JE. Refeeding, metabolic rate, and weight gain in anorexia nervosa: a review. *Int J Eat Disord.* 1995;17(4):337-345.

22. Caggiani C. Using enteral feeding to support eating disorder recovery. *SCAN's Pulse.* 1999:12-14.

23. Woods BK, Runyan B, Lamb RP. Perspectives in nasogastric feeding the eating disorder patient. *Infant Child Adolesc Nutr.* 2009;1:257-261.

24. Sachs K, Andersen D, Sommer J, Winkelman A, Mehler PS. Avoiding medical complications during the refeeding of patients with anorexia nervosa. *Eat Disord.* 2015;9:1-11.

25. Hofer M, Pozzi A, Joray M, et al. Safe refeeding management of anorexia nervosa inpatients an evidence-based protocol. *Nutrition.* 2014;30(5):524-530.

26. Rocks T, Pelly F, Wilkinson P. Nutrition therapy during initiation of refeeding in underweight children and adolescent inpatients with anorexia nervosa: a systematic review of the evidence. *J Acad Nutr Diet.* 2014;114(6):897-907.

27. Agostino H, Erdstein J, Di Meglio G. Shifting paradigms: continuous nasogastric feeding with high caloric intakes in anorexia nervosa. *J Adolesc Health.* 2013;53(5):590-594.

28. Tresley J, Sheean PM. Refeeding syndrome: recognition is the key to prevention and management. *J Am Diet Assoc.* 2008;108(12):2105-2108.

29. Caggiani C. Monitoring enteral feeding to support eating disorder recovery. *SCAN's Pulse.* 1999:10-11.

30. Setnick J. Micronutrient deficiencies and supplementation in anorexia and bulimia nervosa: a review of literature. *Nutr Clin Pract.* 2010;25(2):137-142.

31. FDA backs use of Prozac for bulimia. *New York Times.* November 13, 1994. www.nytimes.com/1994/11/13/us/fda-backs-use-of-prozac-for-bulimia.html. Accessed August 10, 2010.

32. US Food and Drug Administration. FDA expands uses of Vyvanse to treat binge eating disorder [news release]. January 10, 2015. www.fda.gov/NewsEvents/Newsroom/PressAnnouncements/ucm432543.htm. Accessed February 25, 2016.

33. McElroy SL, Arnold LM, Shapira NA, et al. Topiramate in the treatment of binge eating disorder association with obesity: a randomized, placebo-controlled trial. *Am J Psychiatry.* 2003;160:255-261.

34. Stein K. When essential medications provoke new health problems: the metabolic effects of second-generation anti-psychotics. *J Am Diet Assoc.* 2010;110(7):992-1001.

35. American Dietetic Association. Position of the American Dietetic Association: integration of medical nutrition therapy and pharmacotherapy. *J Am Diet Assoc.* 2010;110(6):950-956.

36. Pronsky ZM, Crowe JP. *Food Medication Interactions.* 16th ed. Food Medication Interactions. Birchrunville, PA:2008.

Chapter 5

Nutrition Intervention for Eating Disorders: Nutrition Education

In a general hospital or unit, nutrition education usually takes a back seat to Food and/or Nutrient Delivery, as most eating disorder patients only stay long enough to be stabilized and transferred to a specialty center or psychiatric unit. You may be frustrated that some patients do not change their eating habits on your advice during their brief hospital stay. This is not a reflection on you but a reflection of the severity of the illness and the long course of treatment.

In this setting, nutrition education may be directed more toward caregivers and family members, answering questions and providing or recommending reading materials to help them understand their loved one's condition. If a patient is leaving your hospital for home, rather than an alternate treatment setting, provide a meal plan to the patient and caregiver that will be feasible in the home environment, along with a referral to an outpatient registered dietitian nutritionist (RDN).

Most eating disorder education falls into the comprehensive category and is provided over time in nutrition counseling sessions. In treatment settings where you have opportunities over time to gradually introduce and increase nutrition education, the topics you choose will vary depending on each individual's needs. Eating disorder patients may appear to know plenty of nutrition *information*—facts, Recommended Daily Allowances (RDAs), calorie counts— yet may have little skill in using it for their health.

Many of the nutrition "facts" that these patients use to guide their lives are actually nutrition myths, misconceptions, or misinterpretations that they have gleaned from internet magazines, peers, or diet programs. Some eating disorder rules may have simply been invented, without any grain of nutrition truth behind them.

Nutrition education for eating disorders, therefore, will likely focus on providing basic nutrition information in the context of daily eating, the physical and nutrition-related effects of eating disorders and of nutritional rehabilitation, implementation of nutrition recommendations (such as food shopping and preparation), and long-term nourishment, rather than on calories, fat grams, or individual nutrients. Several key eating disorder-related nutrition education topics are reviewed in the following section.

Principles of Good Nutrition

If a patient has never encountered an RDN before, your first teaching topic will be the role you hope to play and the long-term nature of nutritional recovery. The information about your patient's beliefs and behaviors that you gathered during your assessment informed your creation of an initial meal plan. Because this initial meal plan might not have been nutritionally balanced, your patient or his or her family members may express concern that "this is not normal eating." You may be able to reassure concerned caregivers that the initial meal plan is just a starting point for their loved one's treatment. It is impossible to predict at the beginning of treatment how long a full recovery will take, but eventually your goal is something more balanced and "normal." Although you will be slowly but surely encouraging the patient to expand his or her palate, coercion or bribery from family members to eat foods that are not included in the meal plan is not helpful.

The basic principles of good nutrition provide a clear and logical framework for you to allay the concerns of all involved. Unlike a healthy individual, for whom the

principles as a whole are a guide, your patient must view
the principles as steps, meeting them one at a time and *in
order*. Applied to eating disorder recovery, the principles of
good nutrition build on each other, prioritizing necessities
and presenting a new challenge as each goal is met. Box 5.1
describes the principles of good nutrition and their role in
eating disorder recovery.

Box 5.1 Principles of Good Nutrition for Eating Disorder Recovery	
Principle	Criteria for completion and progression to next principle
1. Adequacy	Intake during waking hours is sufficient to meet *energy* needs of daily living, voluntary physical activity, and weight goals.
2. Balance	Intake includes at least one selection from every food group and is sufficient to meet *macronutrient* needs.
3. Variety	Intake includes several/many/most (as applicable) choices from every food group and is sufficient to meet *micronutrient* needs.
4. Moderation	Intake *does not exceed* recommended quantities of any food, nutrient, or bioactive or nonnutritive substance.
5. Nutrient density	Intake is *primarily* (not exclusively) composed of nutrient-rich foods.
6. Autonomy	Intake is based on *personal preferences* rather than the expectations of others. Nutritional factors are considered in planning meals, rather than weight concerns, obsessions, or irrational beliefs. Regret after eating is manageable and does not result in compensatory behaviors.
7. Confidence	Intake is *spontaneous* and based on internal cues rather than a fixed schedule. Meals do not need to be planned in advance. Decisions can be made in the moment about what, when, and how much to eat. Participation in social and other activities does not revolve around what food will be available. Choices are almost always made without regret.

These principles must be adopted sequentially in order to provide a solid foundation for long-term recovery. An example would be a patient whose meal plan includes eating scrambled eggs several times each day. It's easy to understand why a family member might express concern. The RDN's explanation of the principles of good nutrition for eating disorder recovery provides a base for the family member to understand that the patient is striving to meet *adequate* calorie needs, and that scrambled eggs are one of the few "safe" foods that he or she will eat in a large enough quantity to do so. With gentle guidance and support, the RDN can convey to the family member that scrambled eggs are only the first step in a comprehensive plan to move the patient toward health and confidence.

You may find that an individual fears reaching the confidence stage because he or she believes that it requires giving up all control over food. Reassure your patient that this stage in fact signifies being *in* control of eating and food rather than being controlled *by* them. Confidence is the intersection of good nutrition and intuitive eating. A patient in the confidence stage of recovery does not eat anything and everything: He or she makes choices based on appropriate criteria (hunger level, food availability, likes and dislikes, to name a few) rather than fear. This is also helpful information for family members, who may mistake personal choices (such as declining dessert) for eating disorder behavior.

"Legalizing" Food

An important concept on the path to autonomy in eating is the recognition that although the lifelong goal is "good nutrition," this means a balance over time, not a designation of individual foods as "good" or "bad."[1] Individuals with eating disorders often attribute far too much power to individual foods or ingredients. Foods labeled as bad or unhealthy are given the powers to "ruin the day," make the eater a bad person, cause emotional distress, or somehow compromise the integrity of the individual's eating as a whole. Some patients take these misconceptions a step further, to where eating "bad" foods warrants punishment, purging, or another kind of penance.

Legalizing food describes the process of decriminalizing eating and removing moral qualities and negative powers from food. This returns food to its appropriate status as simply (but so importantly) nourishment for life. Foods are no longer referred to as "good" and "bad" but should be referred to as:

- "more nutritious" or "less nutritious";
- "more to my liking" or "less to my liking"; and
- "unsupportive to my recovery" or "supportive to my recovery."

Legalizing food does not mean giving up all preferences and eating "anything and everything," as many patients fear. It simply takes magical powers away from individual foods and makes all foods "allowed." Especially for patients who have experienced overeating or who for any reason have been forced to eat unwanted foods, this reassurance can be essential. There is a healthy balance to be found between restricting and overeating, where most foods are allowed, eaten in response to hunger, and occasionally even eaten purely for pleasure.

One benefit to legalizing food is that it neutralizes the power of "forbidden" foods.[2] If all foods are allowed, there is less incentive to restrict, binge, purge, or secretly eat. Legalizing food does not mean it *must* be eaten, it only means it *can* be eaten. As Carolyn Costin, author of *The Eating Disorder Sourcebook*,[3] has said, "I don't care if you never eat a brownie again; I just care if you WANT a brownie that you're not AFRAID of it."

Legalizing food begins as a concept and a goal, rather than a behavior. Teach your patient the concept, even if he or she is not yet willing to embrace it. It may takes weeks or more of successful eating experiences before a formerly forbidden food can be eaten without remorse. Because American culture reinforces the good/bad dichotomy of food, patients will be challenged by external messages at the same time they are trying to change their internal ones. If your facility encourages or requires patients to eat "risk" foods or "food challenges," support should be provided before and after for the intense feelings of shame and guilt that may arise, along with the temptations to purge. Some patients will feel shame and guilt not just for eating the food but additionally for *enjoying* it.

Individuals who have restricted themselves from eating some or many foods may need to relearn which foods they actually like and dislike. They may have convinced themselves otherwise based on arbitrary or learned food rules or fears. Recovery presents an opportunity to reevaluate food and beverage preferences and to trial different things and determine which to include in daily life, which to include only occasionally, and which to primarily avoid.

Although eating disorder treatment may require challenges and discomfort, ultimate recovery does not require that a person eat or like every food. The important distinctions between an appropriate food restriction and an eating disordered one are the conscious, purposeful manner in which the decision is made, rather than an impulsive, compulsive, or reactionary manner; and that the motive for the decision is individually determined, rather than based on perceptions of others, mistaken beliefs, or shame.

Weight Issues

Weight is a very compelling issue during eating disorder treatment for many different reasons that you are likely to encounter in the course of your work.

Individuals with eating disorders may be anxious about their body weight and how it may affect their appearance, obsessed with or overreactionary to minute changes in weight and movement up or down, compelled to weigh themselves multiple times each day but petrified of being weighed by others, and ambivalent or fearful about how recovery will influence their weight. As the dietitian, you may be considered the keeper of the weight and therefore the target of questions you cannot answer when your patients are desperate to know what you think their weight should be, how fast they will be expected to gain weight, how quickly they can possibly lose weight, and how you know that their current weight is not just fine as is.

Well-meaning family members may use weight restoration or weight loss as the sole goal of recovery and focus on weight normalization at any cost rather than well-rounded treatment. They may misinterpret weight normalization as a sign that the patient no longer needs treatment or follow-up care. They may express that if the patient could just gain or lose weight that "everything will be okay" or fail to acknowledge successful behavior change if it doesn't result in a desired weight change. They may have their own ideas about what their loved one should weigh that may not agree with your clinical assessment. And they may wonder why you cannot make their loved one's weight go up or down any faster.

Insurance companies often use weight information as the sole determining factor for coverage decisions for eating disorder patients and may deny coverage to patients whose weight is considered normal even though their eating behaviors are life-threateningly severe. Insurance companies sometimes try to terminate treatment early based on unsatisfactory (to them) weight change, even though treatment is clearly effective in other areas.

You may encounter other professionals who will argue with you about what a patient's goal weight should be, or how fast or slow it should proceed. You may disagree about the urgency of a higher level of care in the absence of recommended weight change. Unfortunately there are many professionals (including some dietitians) who believe weight loss is the cure for everything or who treat heavier individuals differently than they would treat a smaller patient with the same condition.

Debating goal weights and goal weight gain or loss rates can be endless, as well as a distraction from the true work of recovery. For all of these reasons, you may at times find it helpful to maintain a weight-neutral stance with regard to nutritional rehabilitation. Focus on nutrition and eating behavior with your patients, their family members, and their treatment team, with weight change as an outcome rather than a goal. A change in a patient's weight provides information and may contribute to health, but it is not the sole determining factor. In many cases, it is not even an important one. This is going to be a challenging concept to convey in our weight-obsessed society.

Educate your patients that "ideal body weight" is a concept, and possibly a faulty one, not one fixed number per person. A true healthy weight is determined by optimal functioning and appropriate vital signs, is influenced by many variables, and changes throughout a lifetime. It is useful to have a goal weight toward which to strive, but the target may change as more information is received during recovery.

An ideal weight is one that can be maintained with appropriate eating and physical activity without purging or other eating disorder behaviors, and one at which blood pressure,

body temperature, heart rate, and reproductive functioning are within normal limits. It takes time in recovery
before weight stabilizes and health is restored. Therefore
it is impossible at the beginning of treatment to determine
a single weight that will cause health. Conversely, weight
alone does not indicate health or recovery. Patients with
bulimia, who often fit into normal weight categories, often
lose weight when they are no longer bingeing or purging.

Avoiding Numbers

Many individuals with eating disorders find that numbers
of any kind are "sticky" and persist in their minds, long
after they are no longer relevant. Examples of numbers that
stick might be the weight a pediatrician recommended for
the patient as a child or the proper weight according to a
chart. As much as possible, avoid discussing weight-related
numbers with patients, including future weight goals, current weight, and weight increases. Patients may become
obsessed with certain numbers, afraid of certain weights,
and may sabotage treatment when nearing a goal weight.
They may fear that reaching a goal weight will symbolize
that they no longer need the support of treatment professionals and family members. Obsessions with weight are
part and parcel of eating disorders, so the best course of
action for the RDN is to limit this type of discussion and
explain that it is not possible to know an exact healthy goal
weight at the outset of treatment. Deeper work with the
mental health professional on the team be required to
identify possible negative attachments to weight and move
beyond them.

Determining Healthy Weight

Recent and past weight history can provide helpful information for estimating healthy weight goals, but the
pre–eating disorder weight is not automatically the goal.

Many individuals develop eating disorders after appropriately initiating weight loss. In other words their usual body weight was high, their current body weight is low, their healthy body weight is somewhere in between. Patients who were formerly very muscular but have lost much of their body mass should not be expected to gain back to their original weight. Even if an individual's former body weight fits within normal parameters for their height and age, that is no guarantee that the patient was a healthy eater. Guide your patient to look ahead toward a "new normal" rather than back to "how things used to be."

Notwithstanding all of the preceding, RDNs are still sometimes asked to provide an ideal body weight for a patient. Because there is no universally accepted standard, you must use the information you have at hand to estimate. Use available anthropometric data and standards along with weight history and clinical judgment to estimate an initial weight goal that may be revised as the patient progresses in recovery and additional data points are available. Body mass index (BMI) is used to designate severity of anorexia nervosa in *Diagnostic and Statistical Manual of Mental Disorders,* fifth edition (*DSM-5*), and it is used in some facilities and by some health insurance companies to determine weight goals. However, using BMI to predict a healthy weight is limited, especially for adults, as it does not discriminate between males and females, body composition, muscle mass or wasting, loss of bone density, and so on. Because of its current popularity of use by governmental entities and others, it is included here, but its use as a standard without also incorporating individual differences and clinical judgment is discouraged.

Weighing Protocol

If you are responsible for gathering anthropometric data on your patient, it will be worth your time to discuss the process beforehand and, as much as possible, honor the patient's preferences of when and how to go about it (eg, beginning vs end of session, in street clothes vs in a gown, facing the numbers vs back to the numbers). If other staff members are responsible for gathering anthropometrics, they should be trained in the special concerns of eating disorder patients and requested to refrain from commenting on the patient's weight status over time as "good/bad" or "better/worse."

As preoccupation with weight and body size is symptomatic of eating disorders, you and other staff members should use caution in sharing anthropometric data with patients. Every piece of information will be viewed through the distorted filter of the eating disorder, so normal or healthy values may be interpreted by the patient as upsetting or unacceptable. If possible, determine a course of action with the other members of your treatment team regarding weighing and measuring each patient and how this information will be discussed with him or her.

If a weighing protocol is not already in place at your facility, the following general guidelines can be used as a guide for training:

- Individuals with eating disorders should be weighed in private, apart from other patients. Patient weights should not be discussed in group sessions even if a patient is comfortable with his or her weight, as the numbers and their inevitable comparisons may be triggering to other patients.
- Avoid comments, even compliments, about a patient's weight. "Good job! You gained a pound!" can trigger eating disorder thoughts and behaviors in a patient who has mixed feelings about this aspect of recovery.
- Discourage patients and family and staff members from considering weight to be good, bad, or even a sign that the patient is doing well or doing worse. Instead,

consider weight to be simply another vital sign, like heart rate, blood pressure, or temperature, thinking of it as one piece of information that is added to other pieces to paint a complete picture of the situation.

- Discourage staff and family members from commenting on weight as if it were something to be excited or disappointed about, because the patient cannot truly control his or her weight. Outside pressure on a patient to gain or lose weight can tempt him or her to manipulate it by water-loading or by other means. It is acceptable to ask a patient how he or she feels about his or her own weight, rather than to say, "You must be so excited!" or "You must feel disappointed right now."

- Family and staff members should not comment about their own weights in front of patients.

Some individuals may find it helpful (although they may be unwilling at first) to be weighed backward (or with their eyes closed) so that they are unable to monitor daily or insignificant weight fluctuations. Patients whose weights are not in danger may prefer not to be weighed at all and may be encouraged that frequent weighing (contrary to the messages conveyed by American culture) is not essential to healthy weight maintenance. Keep in mind that overweight patients may be just as obsessed with monitoring their body weight as underweight patients. Although family members may claim that an overweight patient doesn't care about his or her weight, this is unlikely. Encourage family members to strive for a weight neutral environment in the home, where weight and weight changes are not discussed.

Weight Gain Guidelines

In higher levels of care, such as a hospital or treatment center, more rapid weight gain can be expected and monitored. Practice guidelines from the American Psychiatric

Association (APA) suggest 2 to 3 pounds of weight gain per week; some treatment centers strive for more. Many factors may influence the rate of weight gain in the inpatient setting, including risk of refeeding syndrome, patient willingness to accept nutrition support, and hypermetabolism (because of the high caloric needs of weight restoration). In outpatient care, weight gain may be slower and less consistent. APA practice guidelines suggest 0.5 to 1 pound per week.[4]

These basic recommendations should be modified depending on your facility's protocol as well as each individual's needs. Modify meal plans on an individual basis by monitoring the pace of weight change. Change meal plans when you see a pattern of data that indicates a patient has reached an appropriate caloric level, rather than on each and every new data point.

Rate of Weight Change

It is unusual for weight gain to follow any exact pattern or to maintain a constant rate over time. This may be disappointing to a patient who wants to recover quickly and move on, but it can be reassuring to a patient who is frightened of rapid changes. Either way, it is a teaching opportunity that weight is a consequence of eating *over time*; one food, one meal, or one day does not have enough power to change everything. Weight loss, weight restoration, and healthy weight maintenance are all long-term, rather than immediate, goals. This may be very different from a patient's usual "quick fix" methods.

At times, weight changes may be dramatic, especially toward the beginning of treatment. When this occurs, teach your patients that quick weight changes are caused by hormone fluctuations, fluid shifts, nutrient replenishment, and the movement of food and beverages through the gastrointestinal (GI) tract, not by the food they ate yesterday.

Discourage patients from attempting to determine exactly which food caused which weight change.

When a patient's weight changes unexpectedly or does not change when a patient hoped it would, reassure your patient that he or she is not a disappointment to you. Often eating disorder patients gauge their self-worth and their worth to others by their weight. You can role-model that weight is not relevant to your regard for your patient, and that you are proud of him or her for making the efforts that will ultimately lead to recovery. Focus on improved eating behaviors and weight will follow.

Family Education

Be sure to include concerned family members in your education about weight so that they bring their questions to you rather than to the patient. Encourage them to view recovery as much more than weight restoration or weight loss and to look for other signs of success. Education from you and the other treatment team members may be needed to combat the common misconception (or wishful thinking) of patients and family members that weight restoration or achievement of a healthy weight constitutes a full recovery. Emphasize that mental and physical recovery must continue even after weight normalization, otherwise the risk of relapse is great. If a patient perceives that once weight is restored, he or she will no longer receive "special treatment," attention, or needed mental health care, he or she may sabotage treatment in order to "stay sick." This is referred to as "secondary gain." If you believe that this is happening, share your concerns with the family therapist or other mental health professional on the team.

Physical Activity

Physical activity guidelines for an individual with an eating disorder should be made by the treatment team based on the patient's physical stability and health, current nutrition intake, and past history of exercise compulsivity.[5] When a patient is medically cleared to exercise, educate him or her about the energy cost of daily living, the additional energy needs of exercise, and how to modify the meal plan to meet these additional needs.

Underweight patients may be allowed to exercise with supervision, as long as weight gain continues at an appropriate pace. However, exercise is not always appropriate; if a patient is unable to consume adequate calories to support activities of daily living, extra activities should not be allowed. Patients should be advised to stop exercising immediately and report to their physician or emergency room if they experience chest pain, shortness of breath, muscle weakness, dizziness, heart palpitations, fatigue, heat intolerance, or other signs of distress.

Individuals who have compulsively exercised as a purging method and competitive athletes who have never experienced exercise in a leisurely manner may need to trial different types of exercise to determine one or more activities they actually enjoy. Encourage noncompetitive, social, or meditative forms of exercise, such as yoga, Pilates, dance, or leisure walks. Competition and team sports should be avoided until much later in recovery, as patients may find it difficult to respect their physical limitations or respond to signs of fatigue when competing or when they think others are relying on their performance.

Purging: Vomiting, Laxatives, and Diuretics

Although purging does not "work" as a weight-loss tool, patients feel lighter and emptier after vomiting or using laxatives, as well as a sense of relief. They may be surprised to find that this does not necessarily mean they have lost weight or body mass. Education regarding the harmful effects of purging on the GI tract and overall health and nutrition status is important, although it is not often adequate to change behavior.[4]

Even patients who have quit "cold turkey" from nicotine or other addictions may be surprised how difficult they find resisting the urge to purge. Help them understand the compulsive nature of these behaviors and that medication may be necessary to help them stop. If a patient can resist the urge to purge, it may dissipate. Supervision or support from family members for a set amount of time after meals, either in person, by phone, or on the Internet, may be essential. Work with the mental health professional on the team to determine other appropriate, helpful distractions.

Vomiting

Discourage patients from brushing their teeth immediately after vomiting, as this can further erode and damage tooth enamel beyond the effects of the stomach acid itself. Rinsing with baking soda and water will neutralize the acid and mitigate damage to the teeth. Patients whose teeth hurt when eating, drinking, or vomiting should be evaluated by a dental professional, as cavities and infection are common. An infection that enters the bloodstream or bone of the jaw can be severe. Discourage patients from using foreign objects to induce vomiting, as these can be a choking hazard. A patient who has accidentally swallowed a toothbrush or other implement should seek emergency care, as this may require surgical removal. If a patient observes blood when vomiting, a physician should be consulted. This can be minor, as in broken esophageal blood vessels, or major, as in perforation of the esophageal wall.

Trigger Foods

If an individual can identify certain foods, such as binge foods or trigger foods that are known to cause inevitable urges to purge, advise him or her to avoid those foods for the time being. It is preferable for a patient to eat and keep down a nutritionally unbalanced meal rather than eating and purging one with "perfect" nutrition. Ipecac syrup, used to induce vomiting in cases of accidental poison ingestion, can be fatal if used repeatedly, as it builds up in a patient's body over time. A patient who refuses to give up using ipecac should be hospitalized. If a patient is genuinely unable to keep down any food or fluids or is unable to decrease the frequency of purging behaviors, consider a higher level of care where the patient can be more closely monitored and supported.

Laxatives

The assortment of laxative products available over the counter is astounding. Add to that the number of foods and beverages with a known or intended laxative effect, and the potential for abuse is obvious. Although laxative abuse is not an effective weight-loss tool, it does provide a cleansing, empty feeling that can lead to a sense of relief after eating, and over time to psychological or physiological dependence. Laxative abuse can result from a genuine need that spirals out of control. It can also develop solely as a part of the eating disorder.

It is very unusual for an individual who abuses laxatives to stop "cold turkey" unless hospitalized, and rebound constipation is possible. There is no professional agreement on a weaning process for laxative abuse. A GI evaluation by a physician skilled in eating disorder treatment is advised for any patient with a history of laxative abuse. Permanent damage to the GI tract, occasionally leading to cathartic colon and the need for surgery, can occur.

In cases where a laxative is genuinely needed to promote bowel function, the physician should provide detailed guidelines for appropriate use. If an individual is not able to follow this prescription, a supportive family member or nurse (depending on the level of care) should store the medication and distribute the appropriate dose at the appropriate time. A psychiatric evaluation is also indicated because of the psychological nature of the dependence; a patient can become extremely anxious when attempting to decrease his or her reliance on what he or she perceives to be an effective weight gain prevention tool. Behavioral interventions by the mental health professional will likely be required as well.

The RDN's role in the weaning process is largely educational. Topics you may cover include:

- the ineffectiveness of laxatives as weight management tools;
- the process in which laxatives actually effect the GI tract only after food has mostly been digested;
- the potential dangers of continued use;
- the length of time that is normal for food to travel the digestive tract under natural conditions; and
- recommended intake of fluid and fiber, including types of fiber. Fiber supplementation should be approved by the physician prior to recommendation by the RDN.

Food Procurement and Preparation

The proliferation of basic cookbooks teaching "how to boil water" and "how to cook an egg" attest to the lack of food preparation skill of many adults today. Some individuals with eating disorders are unequipped to independently nourish themselves, while others are very proficient in the kitchen, cooking and baking food for others while they refuse to feed themselves. For patients in the former category, your educational goals may include grocery shopping, purchasing and learning to use needed kitchen tools and supplies, learning to follow a recipe and safely use appliances, food safety and storage, and food preparation techniques before you even advance to the stage of making an actual meal.

This may seem painfully simplistic, especially if you are an accomplished cook yourself, but keep in mind that a person with an eating disorder is not functioning at his or her full potential. Falling asleep after binge eating while a pot of water boils over on the stove or cross-contaminating utensils are potentially dangerous scenarios that can easily occur unless strategies are in place to prevent them.

Education in situ is especially helpful if you have the opportunity. Grocery shopping and cooking with patients, individually or in a group, can help decrease the anxiety threshold that makes these activities so intimidating. Meal management, recipe reading, and drawing up a list of needed supplies are tasks that may be completely new. Even if a patient does not wish to eat a food that has been prepared together, encounters with food (purchasing, smelling, touching, observing others eating) helps build the skills needed for recovery. Discuss with a patient in advance his or her (perceived) barriers to home food preparation, and you are likely to hear anything from "I don't know what to buy" to "I don't want anyone at the grocery store to know I eat." Every barrier has an alternative, with the one exception of "I just don't want to." If a patient is not willing to prepare his or her own food, then the timing simply is not right. There are other ways to stay nourished without having to learn to cook.

Restaurants and Other Social Settings

While some individuals are unequipped to prepare their own meals and prefer eating out or "ordering in," others much prefer the comfort and control of eating only their own foods. While this may be effective and adequate in the early stages of recovery, eventually most patients will encounter the need to eat in public. This may occur as a wish to be "more normal"—eat in a restaurant, go to a friend's house for dinner, attend a party—in which case there is an opportunity to plan ahead what to eat, problem-solve tricky situations that may arise, and practice with a support person (possibly you). Education may include:

- "portion distortion" (when restaurants serve large portions) and how to manage it (share an entree, order an appetizer and a salad, and so forth);
- social and self-care skills (such as asking the server to remove a complimentary bread basket or looking up a menu online in advance);
- the downside of saving up for 1 or more days in order to splurge at a party; and
- backup strategies (bringing a snack in case there is no acceptable food available when needed, and so forth).

Special Events

Other situations are less predictable and more stressful, even without the added stress of the eating aspect, such as a first date, meeting a significant other's parents, or participating in a wedding, performance, or reunion. In addition to your help with the eating piece of these events, the patient may benefit from consultation with the mental health professional on the team for stress management and problem-solving techniques for social stressors that may arise. Body image issues can flare up in advance of an event in which your patient must stand in front of a group, and the temptations of eating disorder behaviors will be strong. If your patient turns to alcohol in social situations or to handle stress, taking into account that alcohol alters one's judgment regarding what and how much to eat may influence the eating plan. In extremely stressful or hostile situations, you may suggest that your patient plan not to eat at the event at all but to modify the meal plan before and after the event instead. If the anxiety in advance of an event is not manageable with appropriate planning and problem solving, a psychiatric evaluation may be helpful in identifying a possible social anxiety disorder and corresponding treatment.

Prevention

You may be asked for an opinion on whether eating disorders can be prevented. Epigenetic research suggests that eating disorder development is related in almost equal parts to genetic predisposition (nature) and environmental triggers (nurture),[5] however the impact of each contribution is multifactorial. Box 5.2 lists suggested methods for decreasing the environmental load that encourages eating disorder development. Once an eating disorder has been set in motion, the most crucial dimension is obtaining care. Care should never be delayed by a parent or caregiver who fears being blamed for a child or other family member's eating disorder.

Although it is unclear the degree to which societal factors actually cause eating disorders, it is blatantly obvious that the American obsession with weight, fitness, dieting, and food conceals many eating disorders until they are very severe. However, at the time of this writing, the cultural milieu in the United States appears to be undergoing the very beginnings of change regarding acceptance of diversity in body shape and size.

Dieting very rarely leads to lasting weight loss; each failed diet is simply replaced by a newer version. Dieters gain back lost weight, only to blame themselves rather than the impossible-to-follow diet pattern. More recently, increasing awareness of the dangers of dieting itself, even dieting that does not lead to a diagnosable eating disorder, has bolstered the "non-diet" or "health at any size" movement. Spreading the word that dieting is not effective and can be harmful may contribute to the decrease of new cases of eating disorders over time.

Box 5.2 Strategies to Reduce the Risk of Eating Disorder Development

1. Do not make disparaging comments on weight, body shapes or what you or someone else is eating.

2. Do not keep a bathroom scale and only weigh children at their medical checkups.

3. Guide children to follow their own bodies' signals for when, what, and how much to eat. Teach them to say "No, thanks" to food that is offered when they're not hungry.

4. When children or teens announce decisions to change their eating, always ask why. Listen for any ulterior motive that is not food related, such as, "So I'll have more friends," or "So I'll do better in school." Teach healthy methods of handling these situations. Ask the school counselor if you are unsure what to say.

5. When a child you know is feeling down or disappointed, encourage healthy methods of expression, such as talking, writing, or art, rather than eating or dieting.

6. Teach media literacy. Explain that the images we see on billboards and in print are modified by computer to appear unreal. It is not reasonable to compare our own bodies to these standards.

7. Seek professional help for any child or teen who appears to be struggling with weight loss or gain, body image, or eating. If needed, seek help for yourself in order to be a better role model for healthy eating and body image.

References

1. Tribole E. Intuitive eating in the treatment of eating disorders: the journey of attunement. *Renfrew Perspect.* 2010(Winter):11-14.

2. Tribole E, Resch E. *Intuitive Eating: A Revolutionary Program That Works.* 2nd ed. New York: St. Martin's Griffin; 2003.

3. Costin C. *The Eating Disorder Sourcebook: A Comprehensive Guide to the Causes, Treatments and Prevention of Eating Disorders.* 2nd ed. Los Angeles: Lowel House; 1996.

4. Yager J, Devlin MJ, Halmi KA, et al. *Practice Guideline for the Treatment of Patients with Eating Disorders.* 3rd ed. Arlington, VA: American Psychiatric Association; 2006.

5. Reiter CS, Graves L. Nutrition therapy for eating disorders. *Nutr Clin Pract.* 2010;25:122-136.

Chapter 6

Nutrition Intervention for Eating Disorders: Nutrition Counseling

Counseling Strategies and Techniques Used in Nutrition Counseling

Motivational Interviewing

The success of many of your interventions will rely heavily on the patient's willingness to work toward recovery, confidence that change is achievable, and ability to persevere in the face of difficulties that will no doubt arise. This is often described as readiness for change, part of the transtheoretical model.[1]

Motivational interviewing (MI) is a counseling technique that assesses this readiness in an attempt to improve an individual's motivation to change and help him or her shift from precontemplative, contemplative, and preparation stages into action.[2] MI techniques include active and reflective listening, open-ended questions, affirmation, and summarization, all of which are appropriate in nutrition counseling.[3]

As long as an individual remains medically stable, MI can be used, even if progress seems stagnant or painfully slow. If a patient is medically or psychiatrically unstable, MI may be unhelpful or may need to be used in a safe setting, such as a higher level of care. When a patient is so malnourished or hostile that he or she cannot think rationally, discussing his or her motivation to change can become impossible, irrelevant, or both.

At times you will encounter a person who believes he or she is ready to change but is unable to follow through with your recommended intervention(s). This does not mean that you must stop working with the patient. If you think that continuing to meet with the patient will put you or the patient in danger, then discontinuing your care is appropriate. But if the patient is simply taking longer to change than what you or family members predicted or hoped for, it is helpful to adjust your (and, if possible, their) expectations, continuing to work with the individual on his or her terms.

In some cases, motivation to change is high but confounded with an equal or greater reluctance to change. MI by the registered dietitian nutritionist (RDN) can explore this ambivalence on the surface level of food and eating behaviors, but when it stems from fear of failure and other emotional issues, it must be addressed by the mental health professional. Focusing solely on food interventions can be appealing to the patient, as it is distracting from more painful, existential issues, but it prevents true recovery. It is wise to consult with other treatment team members, a trusted colleague, or a supervisor in these situations to help you evaluate whether to push the patient to attempt eating interventions or to support the patient in maintaining the status quo until barriers to action have been addressed in therapy. Explain to the patient and family that conscious motivation and desire are not the only factors in eating disorder recovery, just as weight restoration and balanced eating are not the only goals.

Coping Skills

If patients can see that their eating disorders are harmful, then why is that not motivation enough to change? In addition to the mood-stabilizing chemical changes that eating disorder behaviors offer, they also provide temporary relief (distraction or escape) from the stresses of life. Eating disorders start for many different reasons. They continue, for one: They seem to work. Eventually the original behaviors no longer provide the desired response. Individuals must restrict more, binge more, purge more, and exercise more to achieve the same outcome they originally received. Eventually the reason behind the disorder moves completely from consciousness, and it simply becomes a habitual behavior removed from reason.

Cognitive Behavioral Therapy

To heal from an eating disorder, replacement techniques must be implemented that provide the same benefits as the negative behaviors. If the disorder developed in response to developmental transitions, then those transitions must be navigated in some other way. If the disorder developed because of feelings of inadequacy and low self-esteem, then those must be addressed. If the eating disorder provides escape from unwanted tasks, then that must be provided in another form or fashion. Why give up the tool unless you have another one ready to use? Finding this alternate tool is the goal of cognitive behavioral therapy (CBT).

CBT is based on the concept that behaviors are learned and can be unlearned with practice. It is the most thoroughly studied counseling technique in nutrition therapy and in the treatment of eating disorders.[3] Nutrition interventions in the early stages of treatment may not relate to motivation, but they will require coping skills. As nutrition interventions progress, higher calorie foods are introduced, weight increases or decreases, and the level of care changes, additional coping skills will be necessary.[4]

Simply improving eating behaviors without challenging the internal eating disorder environment cannot be considered a true recovery.[5] The most useful question the RDN can ask after a patient agrees to a new intervention is, "What will you do with your feelings afterward?"

We know that breaking an eating disorder rule or habit will feel miserable. We know there are powerful underlying barriers to change. We know that changing behaviors is necessary to survival. The question is how to mediate the negative thoughts and feelings that occur in recovery without resorting once again to harmful eating disorder behaviors.

Planning ahead, problem solving, role playing imaginary situations, and devising a list of supportive activities and people are all strategies that dietitians can use. The RDN can assist the patient both with external strategies (stay out of the bathroom for 1 hour post meals) and internal strategies (remind yourself that you know people who eat cream cheese who are not overweight).

Legalizing food and nutrition education can also be used in CBT. A foundational premise of CBT is the theory that *events* do not cause feelings, *thoughts* about events cause feelings. Related to food, this means that contrary to a patient's belief, eating pizza does not cause guilt. It is the mistaken belief that pizza is bad and causes heart disease and weight gain that causes the guilt. A rule has been created (eg, "Pizza is not allowed.") in an attempt by the patient to avoid not only heart disease and weight gain but also the *feeling of guilt itself*.

Using CBT principles, you can help your patient identify the many thoughts and feelings that drive the eating disorder cycle. You provide education to counteract inaccurate beliefs about food, while the counselor addresses the patient's desire to eliminate all negative feelings. Just because you teach your patient how to incorporate pizza without gaining weight does not mean that he or she will not feel guilt after eating it (or for some patients, just *thinking* about eating it). But recognition that it is the outdated thoughts and beliefs that cause the guilt, *not* the innocent piece of pizza, is a rational (and accurate) point of view rather than a fear-based one. The short-term goal is for the patient to eat a piece of pizza and successfully handle the guilty feelings that result; the long-term goal is to separate guilt from the experience of food.

Dialectical Behavior Therapy

Dialectical behavior therapy (DBT) was developed from CBT by Marsha Linehan, PhD, ABPP, to help individuals with self-harming and suicidal behaviors identify their destructive thoughts without acting on them. DBT is taught in many eating disorder treatment settings as a way to interrupt the path from thoughts to behaviors.

A foundational principle of DBT is that the professional role-models for the patient accepting his or her thoughts and feelings while pointing out other options. This is an easy fit for RDNs as we are taught to align with a patient in a nonjudgmental manner, identify multiple possibilities for how to reach a goal, and assist the patient in determining which method to try.

The four core strategies of DBT are mindfulness, distress-tolerance, emotion regulation, and interpersonal effectiveness. Emotion regulation and interpersonal effectiveness are primarily in the realm of a psychotherapist, however, RDNs teach mindfulness and distress-tolerance concepts frequently and possibly without realizing we are doing so. Mindfulness is the goal when we ask patients to listen for and identify their physical sensations of hunger and satiety, their cravings, and the nonhunger feelings that trigger their eating behaviors. Distress tolerance is the skill needed to resist the urge to exercise inappropriately, purge, or throw away a meal because no one is looking. Finding an alternate activity to "live through" the temptation requires accepting that the urge exists but choosing not to act on it.

Using DBT effectively requires training and practice. RDNs can benefit from learning more about the DBT skills and strategies that can be used to decrease the frequency of destructive eating behaviors. An offshoot of DBT that is also used in eating disorder treatment is acceptance and commitment therapy (ACT). The beauty of nutrition counseling is that is does not require adherence to one specific counseling theory but can pull the most pertinent concepts from any and all sources. As long as you remain within your scope by using these treatment strategies in the service of food, eating, nutrition, and related topics, you are providing appropriate and even exceptional patient care.

Other Counseling Theories

As you continue to learn about eating disorders, counseling techniques and psychotherapy, you will encounter many other types of therapeutic tools and theories used in the treatment of eating disorders. These include rational emotive behavior theory, emotion acceptance behavior therapy, cognitive remediation therapy, family systems theory, psychodrama, eye movement desensitization therapy, bio- and neurofeedback, exposure therapy, integrative cognitive-affective therapy, equine-assisted therapy (using horses), expressive therapy (art, drama, music, dance), and many, many more. Dietitians do not necessarily practice these therapies; in many cases they require special training, credentials, and equipment. But as an eclectic form of therapy, nutrition counseling can pull from a variety of sources to facilitate behavior change and healing.[6-9]

Staying Within Your Scope of Practice

Conversations about body weight, ideal weight, weight loss, and weight gain may fall on both sides of the dietitian–therapist line. American culture portrays weight and appearance changes as solutions for many unrelated issues, and one of our strengths as RDNs is knowing what nutrition can and cannot change. Nutrition counseling incorporates a sifting process, where you may delve into a topic that appears to be nutrition related on the surface, such as unwanted weight gain, and then recognize a nonnutrition issue at its core, such as self-esteem. When you realize that an individual is seeking a nutrition solution for a nonnutrition problem, provide the best care by communicating with the mental health professional on the team and determining how to coordinate and best use each of your skill sets.

It is typical for an RDN working in a counseling setting to wonder if he or she is crossing some kind of imaginary line into mental health professional territory.[10,11] This is a healthy sign of self-awareness and your desire to stay within your ethical scope of practice. Although it may seem to be a blurry line, there is a very distinct category of topics that delineates the scope of the RDN, which is anything that relates to or influences food or eating.[6] As long as conversations with your patients focus primarily on these topics, with the addition of appointment-related matters and polite conversational topics, you are working within your scope.

Guiding the Conversation

If a topic that seems unrelated to food and eating arises, do not panic. Simply guide the conversation to food with a question: "How do you think that affected your eating?" Many situations that are not about food on the surface have some connection to nutrition or eating, especially for an individual working to heal from an eating disorder.

There are some topics that genuinely do not relate to eating or nutrition or where you have handled the nutritional aspects but further help is needed for the core issue. You may think that you have erred in some way when a patient asks you a nonnutrition question or shares a problem that is out of your scope. It is normal to think something like, "What have I done wrong to make this patient think that I am the right person to talk with about this?" To the contrary, when a patient tells you his or her private thoughts, this is an indication that you have done a fine job building rapport and nonjudgmental trust.[7] However, it is not within the scope of your practice to respond with advice on personal issues such as relationships, past trauma or abuse, or other personal topics. In these situations, the appropriate reply is "That would be a great topic to discuss with your counselor."

In some cases, a patient may not be in contact with a counselor when he or she begins working with you. Many patients will seek the services of an RDN thinking that their issues have their root in nutrition, not realizing there is more to the picture. You may be the very first person in whom a patient has confided his or her struggles. In these cases, you are offering a gift to your patients in the form of a sensitive and caring referral to the appropriate psychotherapist or other mental health professional. A simple way to phrase this recommendation is, "I can see that this is an important area for you to discuss, but I'm not the best person to advise you on this issue. I would like to add a counselor to our team." Chapter 7 contains more information about referring a patient to additional types of care.

Keeping the Focus on Nutrition

If you develop a good working relationship with an individual, you may find that conversations flow toward and then away from nutrition-related topics. It is essential to find the right balance between nutrition counseling and chitchat, but it takes time. Remember for most eating disorder patients, you are one of only a few people who have access to very personal details, so when coming in from the outside world, your patients may need time to transition from small talk to serious business. If small talk or "How was your week?" responses start to take up too much of your allotted time, validate the importance of the event to the patient, and then use a transitional phrase to move the topic onto nutrition. Here are some examples:

- "That's so interesting!…I'm curious how that affected your eating."
- "Oh, that's a bummer!…I wonder how that might have turned out differently if you didn't have an eating disorder?"
- "I'm so glad you had that experience!…Tell me—did it make a difference in your eating?"
- "That does sound like a great weekend!…Do you think your eating disorder played a role in how it turned out?"

And if your attempts at transitioning gently are not effective:

- "I've enjoyed hearing about that (or I'm sorry to hear about that)….I would like to hear more, but I'm concerned that we won't have time left for what we need to cover. Can we switch over to nutrition and your meal plan?"

Once in a while, you may meet with a patient who is experiencing very strong feelings. These feelings may or may not be eating disorder related. If they are related ("I'm devastated that I can't go to college because of my eating disorder!"), you may be able to use a transitional phrase, such as the preceding ones, or channel the conversation onto what can be done to advance recovery, and always remember to first offer validation ("That stinks!…I know you will eventually kick this eating disorder and get to college. Let's fight back and show it who's boss! Show me your food diary.")

Other strong feelings are not at all related to the eating disorder and are simply overpowering ("My Grandpa died. I leave tomorrow for his funeral. I am devastated!"). These feelings defy any transitional phrase or channeling of conversation. You are left with two options to offer the patient (always remembering to validate): "That's awful! I'm so sorry to hear about your grandfather. Do you want to have a session with me, or would your time be better used getting ready for your trip?"

Support your patient on whichever choice he or she makes. Some patients cannot focus in times like these, and others prefer a distraction such as nutrition. If you think that your patient is trying to please you by staying when he or she really wants or needs to leave, you may pull rank and say, "I can tell you want to want to stay, but that you really want [or need] to leave. I support you in leaving, it won't hurt my feelings, and we can pick up where we left off when you come back." It is always wise to convey some information to the other treatment team members about the strong feelings, your knowledge of the situation that prompted them, and your decision to cut short (or not) your session.

Effective Team Communication

Because of the RDN's role as a supportive member of the treatment team, patients and family members may ask for general guidance not always related to nutrition. In most cases, these questions are best directed to a physician or therapist, rather than answered directly. Although such questions can seem like simple requests for your opinion ("Do you think our daughter will be ready to go to college in the fall?"), they are usually more complex and require more thorough discussion. In some circumstances they may even be manipulative attempts to pit team members against each other, and you may be unhappily surprised to hear your words used against you later.

Even under ideal circumstances, your patients and their family members do not seek your advice casually; any opinions you share will be viewed as authoritative because of your role as a member of the treatment team. Therefore it is wise to discuss any requests to make changes to the treatment plan with other team members before offering a definitive decision to patient or family.

At the same time, it is crucial to remember that the patient and family are in crisis and may not be hearing or interpreting information well or accurately. Any time a patient or family member repeats something another provider said or did that sounds irregular, it is wise to double-check the situation with the other provider. This is especially helpful when a patient or family member criticizes another provider or indicates that the other provider criticized you. These are not always conscious efforts to disrupt treatment, but they certainly do.

Keeping Professional Boundaries

In the same way that eating disorders can twist an individual's thinking about food, categorizing each food and each eating episode as "all good" or "all bad," the same type of thinking can also apply to people. It is not unusual for an individual in treatment for an eating disorder to warm up to one member of the treatment team more so than the others. If you are this chosen ally, proceed with caution.

It can feel satisfying, even like an accomplishment when a patient who is generally grumpy cheers up when you enter the room. Just remember that everything is not as simple as it seems. The same person who thinks you're great when you decrease her meal plan today may hate your guts when you increase it tomorrow. You cannot let the patient manipulate you by giving you the cold shoulder or by getting special favors. Most of all, do not believe carte blanche any patient's assertions that another treatment team member is unfair, difficult, or incorrect. Encourage the patient to bring this concern to the person in question, otherwise you are assisting the patient in subverting his or her own recovery. If a patient gives you information from another treatment provider that sounds questionable, always take the time to verify the information directly with the other professional.

It is tempting to relate to an individual in your care, especially if he or she is close to you in age, reminds you of someone you know, grew up in your same hometown, or shares other characteristics with you. It is entirely possible that under different circumstances the two of you would have become friends. But your relationship as patient and RDN cannot move past certain professional boundaries.

It is not unusual for patients to unconsciously diminish the authority of their providers by treating them more like peers or friends. Bringing you a latte, offering to fix you up on a date, calling you by a nickname—all of these are examples of simple ways that a patient may attempt to decrease the power differential between the two of you. It is preferable that you speak with another provider on the team, especially a mental health provider, to gauge the significance of this behavior and the potential harm versus benefits of discussing it with the patient.

In some cases, you may decide to leave it alone, not bringing the attempted boundary violations into conversation but consciously keeping your boundaries and actions professional. In other cases, with the support of your treatment team, you or the therapist may comment to the patient on his or her behavior and express your wishes that your relationship stay strictly professional. When patients are learning new ways of behaving, as they must in order to recover, receiving redirection from you or another member of the treatment team can feel like a rejection that then impairs your working relationship. You should not remain in uncomfortable situations to avoid rocking the boat with a patient. Speaking with another professional (even one who does not know the patient, as in professional supervision or mentoring) is the best way to determine your course of action, whether verbal redirection, intervention from

another member of the treatment team or a supervisor, or
other options.

Working with Patients with Personality Disorders

In some situations, a mental health professional on the team
may determine that an individual with an eating disorder
also has a personality disorder. Personality disorders are
commonly co-occurring with eating disorders but are not
diagnosed as easily because the behaviors are not always
apparent.[12] When a patient in your care is diagnosed with
a personality disorder, it is wise to ask for guidance from
the other members of the team. Although your intention
is not to treat the individual for his or her personality disorder, your nutrition counseling may be influenced by the
patient's particular personality traits.

If patients fail to attend scheduled appointments, do not
pay you the agreed-on fee, are not compliant with recommendations that you think are essential for their safety, or
are threatening to you or your staff, you should most definitely tell the patients that you will not continue to be part
of their treatment team unless certain conditions (that you
specify) are met. Such conversations can feel confron-
tational and even emotional, so keep in mind that setting
these boundaries is an intervention in the best interest of
any patient, and once again seek support from the team, a
colleague, or your supervisor.

Appendix D contains information on additional books
and resources by dietitians to help with counseling skills
for eating disorders. If you are interested in learning more
about the counseling theories described in this chapter, see
the following:

- *Cognitive Behavioral Therapy and Eating Disorders*
  by Christopher Fairburn

- *Cognitive Therapy and the Emotional Disorders* by Aaron Beck
- *Dialectical Behavior Therapy for Binge Eating and Bulimia* by Debra Safer, Christy Telch, Eunice Chen, and Marsha Linehan
- *Motivational Interviewing in the Treatment of Psychological Problems* by Hal Arkowitz, William Miller, Stephen Rollnick, and Henny Westra

References

1. Prochaska JO, Norcross JC, DiClemente V. *Changing for Good: A Revolutionary Six-Stage Program for Overcoming Bad Habits and Moving Your Life Positively Forward.* New York: Avon Books; 1994.

2. Bewell-Weiss C, Carter J. Motivational interviewing in the treatment of eating disorders. *Renfrew Perspect.* 2010;(Winter):4-6.

3. Spahn JM, Reeves RS, Keim KS, et al. State of the evidence regarding behavior change strategies in nutrition counseling to facilitate health and food behavior change. *J Am Diet Assoc.* 2010;110(6):879-891.

4. Kleifield EI, Wagner S, Halmi KA. Cognitive-behavioral treatment of anorexia nervosa. *Psych Clin N Amer.* 1996;19(4):715-737.

5. Crow S. Recovery from eating disorders. *Renfrew Perspect.* 2007;(Winter):1-3.

6. Reiter CS, Graves L. Nutrition therapy for eating disorders. *Nutr Clin Pract.* 2010;25:122-136.

7. Kellogg M. *Counseling Tips for Nutrition Therapists: Practice Workbook.* Vol 1. Philadelphia, PA: Kg Press; 2006.

8. Modugno BY. Behind the food: novel factors influencing behavior and food choices in disordered eating. *SCAN's Pulse.* 2009;28(1):13-16.

9. Kratina K, King NL, Hayes D. *Moving Away from Diets: Healing Eating Problems and Exercise Resistance*. 2nd ed. Denton, TX; Helm Publishing; 2003.

10. Salloff-Coste C, Hamburg P, Herzog D. Nutrition and psychotherapy: collaborative treatment of patients with eating disorders. *Bull Menninger Clin*. 1993;57:504-516.

11. Kellogg M. When and how to refer to psychotherapy. *Weight Manage Matters*. 2008;6(2):14-15.

12. Sansone RA, Levitt JL, eds. *Personality Disorders and Eating Disorders: Exploring the Frontier*. New York: Routledge; 2006.

Chapter 7

Nutrition Intervention for Eating Disorders: Coordination of Care

Communicating with Other Providers

During or prior to your initial assessment, permission to communicate with other treatment providers (including any you recommend) should be requested and obtained. If you work in a facility, this may be handled on behalf of all providers at the time of admission. If you work independently, you will need to gather this permission along with names and contact information. Together with the patient and the patient's family members, these providers and you comprise the treatment team, and all members should be included in major treatment decisions.

After completing your initial assessment, it is wise and courteous to follow up with each of the other treatment team members (either in person or via e-mail, fax, or phone call) to obtain additional information and to provide a summary of your assessment and recommendations. If you work in a facility, "case conferences," rounds, or treatment team meetings are ideal times to share information and confer about treatment plans.

If you work independently, you may have to first assist your patient in locating other providers, and then you and those providers can choose preferred methods of conveying and receiving information. At the beginning of treatment, communication may be frequent. As the patient progresses into recovery, communication may proceed on an as-needed basis (communication only when treatment changes or problems develop) or on a regular (weekly, monthly, per visit) basis. Communication can take place in person, by phone, fax, e-mail, or other agreed-on method.

Essential Members of the Treatment Team

Eating disorder treatment at its most basic includes a physician or psychiatrist, a registed dietitian nutritionist (RDN), and a mental health professional. Some individuals will already have the other members of their treatment team in place by the time of your first meeting. If you work independently, you may be surprised to find how many patients believe their eating disorder is solely a nutritional concern that you will single-handedly solve. Many of these patients may be surprised to hear that you believe they should also consult with a mental health professional.

The rise of neighborhood urgent care centers and the myriad problems with health insurance have resulted in many patients not having a primary care provider. In the best of these situations, you have the opportunity to recommend providers with whom you feel comfortable and with whom you work well. If a patient is limited to the providers who accept his or her health insurance, you may find yourself on a treatment team with someone who is not skilled in eating disorders care. Ideally this practitioner will be open to working closely with you, but in some cases he or she may simply not be able to meet the patient's needs. In many cases, health insurance providers will cover specialists at an in network rate if they do not have a comparable physician on their panel.

Referral to Mental Health Care

Referral to mental health care is an important and often essential step in the treatment of eating disorders.[1] Psychotherapy can take many forms and is provided by a variety of practitioners. Learn the credentials for licensed mental health providers in your state. These may include psychologists, nurses, nurse practitioners, social workers, licensed professional counselors, guidance counselors, youth pastors, ministers, rabbis, chaplains, and others. Depending on each patient's diagnosis and needs, different types of counselors and counseling may be appropriate.

In general, it is helpful if the counselor has some familiarity with eating disorder treatment theories, even if he or she is not exclusively an eating disorder specialist. Some counselors use eclectic techniques, similar to dietitians; others specialize in cognitive behavioral therapy, dialectical behavioral therapy, or other methods helpful in eating disorder recovery. The ideal counselor uses evidence-based treatment and is a good personality match with the patient. A patient may choose to meet with more than one counselor to find a successful match. Box 7.1 summarizes situations and topics for which a mental health counseling referral should be made.

Overcoming Objections to Mental Health Care

You may encounter individuals who disagree with or disapprove of your recommendation to pursue counseling. Other patients may tell you that they have already tried counseling and are not willing to try again. It is wise to explain your rationale for your recommendation, and to allow your patient to express his or her point of view. If the patient is concerned about something specific, you may be able to address those fears directly, for example, "I understand that you didn't have a good experience with a previous counselor. You certainly don't have to go back to that person. There are many other options that I can suggest if you'd like," or "I understand that you don't want to talk about your childhood experiences. That would be a great thing to tell a counselor, as well as what you do want to work on."

Box 7.1 Reasons to Refer to a Mental Health Professional

Diagnosis of psychiatric illness, including eating disorder

Relationship or family problems, recent or past

Difficulty adjusting to a recent life change

Behavior changes as a result of stress or life events

Difficulty caring for self or children and difficulty with activities of daily living

Traumatic event(s), including diagnosis of severe, stigmatizing, or debilitating illness and medical recommendations that change quality of life (eg, bed rest, chemotherapy, insulin shots)

Depression, anxiety, or other overwhelming emotions, whether reported or observed (crying in session, agitation, pacing, anger)

Family member(s) are preoccupied with patient's weight or eating

Sudden change in behavior, mood, or mental state, reported or observed

Inability to change even though patient expresses that change is desired

Fears, anxiety, stress, whether warranted or unwarranted, about the course of the eating disorder or recovery

---

Encourage your patient to consider an evaluation of a new therapist as an interview and to try more than one therapist if needed to find a good match. Box 7.2 lists suggests ways to encourage your patient to seek mental health care (see page 164).

When an individual simply refuses to agree to try a counselor, you have three options:

1. Keep a running list of topics you think would benefit from counseling. Keep it in your patient's chart and mention every time a topic comes up that you add to the list. This will show the patient three things: that these are the type of topics appropriate for counseling, that you are not intending to discuss these topics, and that there really are things to talk about with a counselor. It

---

Box 7.2 Overcoming Objections to Mental Health Care

Specify which issues you are recommending for counseling, rather than making a general recommendation for therapy or counseling. For example, to a patient who is overwhelmed with commitments, "I think this counselor could really help you with time management."

To a patient who says, "But I really like talking with you. I don't understand why you want me to see someone else," respond with, "I agree we've done a lot together, and I'm glad that you feel comfortable talking with me, but in this case, I'm not the best person to give you advice. I'd like to help you find a counselor you feel just as comfortable with."

To a patient who doesn't see how a counselor can help, you might say, "We have been working together for a while on this issue, and in my experience, when someone wants to change and can't, there is often something behind it. A counselor is the type of person who can help you find that stumbling block so that our work together will succeed."

To a patient who resists seeing a counselor because "things are going fine right now," suggest 1 visit, just as a backup plan: "Things are going great now, and I'm glad, but I'm concerned that eventually there will be drama again. So right now, while life is nice and calm, check out a couple of therapists and see who you like. Just go once or twice to get to know them a little. That way when crisis hits, you won't be flipping through the yellow pages trying to find someone."

---

is up to you how long you keep this up until you move to the next step.

2. Set a time limit, for example, "I understand you are hesitant about seeing a counselor and you feel that my help is enough to get through this problem. Let's make a deal. Let's give ourselves 3 weeks to keep at it, and when we reevaluate, if things aren't better, you will agree to meet with a counselor." If at the appointed time your patient still refuses, you are left with the last resort.

"We have come to a point where continuing to meet will not move things forward. I have to insist that before we set our next appointment, you have at least one meeting with a counselor. After that meeting, have your counselor call me, and then we will get back together and keep pressing on." The patient may still resist and may not see a counselor. But the boundary you set is a nutrition intervention. You have made a referral, and your patient must choose to pursue recovery or not. If you feel that you are abandoning your patient, or giving up on him or her, speak with a support person about these completely normal feelings. Making a recommendation to help an individual is most certainly not an abandonment, but because you are refusing to meet again, it can definitely feel that way. It is important to get perspective and also to allow yourself to grieve that your patient is struggling.

Supplementary Members of the Treatment Team

Depending on an individual's symptoms and needs, over the course of treatment, a variety of additional support may be added, either for evaluation and consultation, or on an ongoing basis. Table 7.1 (pages 166–168) includes potential team members to whom you may refer your patients. Generally it is appropriate to consult with or inform other members of the treatment team before or after making a referral for additional care.

Discharge and Transfer to a New Setting

At some point, most individuals will be ready to transition from your care. Transitions occur when a patient leaves for college, moves to a new town, or simply wishes to change providers, but by far the most common transition for eating disorder patients is from a hospital or treatment center to a

Table 7.1 Supplementary Treatment Team Members

Team Member	Role	Indication
Psychiatrist or psychiatric nurse practitioner	Evaluation, diagnosis, medication management	Any eating disorder or psychiatric diagnosis
Dentist	Dental care	Chronic vomiting Bruxism (teeth grinding) Gum disease and tooth loss due to malnutrition
Family therapist	Provide support to patient in communicating and improving relationships with family members	Family members argue during or about nutrition counseling Family dynamics contribute to or perpetuate eating disorder behavior Family members not coping well with stress
Physical therapist, exercise physiologist, personal trainer or other movement therapist	Exercise prescription Injury rehabilitation Stress management, relaxation, release of physical tension	Patient has been medically approved to exercise Patient is recovering from injury Patient unaware of appropriate intensity/duration/mode of physical activity
Art therapist	Emotional access and healing through creative expression	Difficulty with self-expression in talk therapy

Continued on next page.

Continued on next page.

Table 7.1 (cont.) Supplementary Treatment Team Members

Team Member	Role	Indication
Religious leader	Spiritual healing	Religious beliefs or conflict with God/Higher Power impairing recovery History of religious abuse (religion used as weapon of guilt or shame in childhood)
Cardiologist	Cardiac care Medical clearance for physical activity	Chest pain, palpitations, shortness of breath Rapid or significant weight loss History or family history of heart disease
Endocrinologist	Hormone evaluation Insulin resistance Diabetes management	Irregular menstrual cycle not attributed to malnutrition Failure to achieve menarche by 17 years Significant weight gain at menarche or menopause Infertility Diagnosis or potential symptoms of diabetes, hypo- or hyperthyroidism, polycystic ovary syndrome (PCOS), or other endocrine disorder

Table 7.1 (cont.) Supplementary Treatment Team Members

Team Member	Role	Indication
Gastroenterologist	Digestive care	Chronic vomiting or laxative abuse Blood in stool or vomit Chronic or severe unexplained abdominal pain Reflux Diagnosis or symptoms of celiac, Crohn's, or irritable bowel diseases Chronic or severe constipation
Speech therapist or speech pathologist	Feeding evaluation	Difficulty chewing or swallowing food or beverages Repeated choking Aversion to eating after surgery or procedure
Group therapist	Support group leader	Poor social support network Desire for peer interaction

community-based setting and vice versa. The decision to change the level of care is usually made by the physician and other members of the treatment team, but also can be informed by the patient, family member(s), and in some unfortunate cases, the health insurance provider. The typical levels of care recognized in eating disorder treatment are outlined in the following section.

Levels of Care in Eating Disorder Treatment

Outpatient Care: Individual appointments are made with care providers in an office or clinic setting. Patients appropriate for this level of care are:

- medically stable and in at least fair general health, requiring infrequent monitoring of weight or vital signs;
- self-motivated toward recovery and in a stable and supportive living environment;
- able to travel to and from scheduled appointments safely and reliably;
- able to follow a meal plan at home or school (100% compliance not required);
- able to resist purging, exercise, and self-harm triggers at home (100% compliance not required); and
- not actively suicidal.

Intensive Outpatient Program: Group meetings are supervised by care providers in 2- to 4-hour increments several times a week. Patients appropriate for this level of care are:

- medically stable and at least in fair general health but possibly requiring weight or vital signs to be monitored more than once per week,
- self-motivated toward recovery and in a stable and supportive living environment,

- able to travel to and from group and individual meetings safely and reliably,
- able to follow a meal plan at home or school (100% compliance not required),
- able to resist purging, exercise, and self-harm triggers at home (100% compliance not required), and
- not actively suicidal.

Day Treatment: This is also called full-day outpatient care or partial hospitalization. Individual and group treatment is offered for the majority of waking hours most days of the week, including one or more supervised meals each day. Day treatment programs may operate during typical work or school hours, such as 8 AM to 4 PM Monday through Friday. Partial hospitalization typically refers to spending 7 days a week in a hospital treatment program, including all meals, but returning home to sleep. Patients appropriate for this level of care are:

- medically stable to leave the hospital or facility but requiring weight or vital signs to be monitored daily,
- having difficulty following a meal plan without supervision at mealtimes,
- having difficulty resisting purging or self-harm triggers without supervision,
- self-motivated enough in treatment to attempt to avoid detrimental behaviors when unsupervised at home in a stable living environment,
- able to travel to and from the facility safely and reliably, and
- not actively suicidal.

Residential Treatment or Treatment Center: Sometimes referred to as "Rehab," it is a freestanding treatment facility that may or may not be affiliated with a hospital and may or may not be devoted exclusively to eating disorders care. Patients appropriate for this level of care are:

- medically compromised and requiring daily or constant monitoring of weight or vital signs;
- unable to travel safely or reliably to treatment;
- in an unstable or unsupportive living environment;
- unable to follow a meal plan without supervision and external motivation;
- unable to resist purging or self-harm triggers without supervision and external motivation and so require supervision using the bathroom; and
- resistant or uncooperative in recovery, requiring constant structure and external motivation to remain safe.

Inpatient Hospitalization: Full hospital care is offered in either a medical, psychiatric, or eating disorders unit. Patients appropriate for this level of care are:

- medically unstable and requiring daily or constant monitoring of weight, vital signs, or laboratory tests, including:
  - heart rate <40 beats per minute (adult) or <50 beats per minute (child/adolescent)
  - blood pressure <90/60 mm Hg (adult) or <80/50 mm Hg (child and adolescent)
  - >10 to 20 mm Hg drop in blood pressure from sitting to standing position
  - glucose level <60 mg/dL
  - potassium <3 mEq/L
  - temperature <97°F
  - dehydrated, hypokalemic or hypophosphatemic, or experiencing hepatic, renal, or cardiovascular complications requiring acute treatment[2]
- malnourished or refusing oral intake, possibly requiring nutrition support;

- weighing < 75% of expected weight in adults or refusing food or experiencing acute weight loss in children, even if weight is within normal limits;
- purging or self-harming unless constantly supervised and may be actively suicidal and may secretly exercise if left unsupervised and requires supervision using the bathroom;
- resistant or uncooperative in recovery, requiring constant structure and external motivation to remain safe, actively attempting to sabotage medical/nutritional care; and
- requiring inpatient hospitalization even if not medically unstable because they are psychiatrically impaired or chemically dependent.

"Step-down" Care, Transitional Living, "Halfway" House, or Group Home: After leaving inpatient or residential treatment, patients may participate in a less-structured living situation intended to prepare them to return to their own home and outpatient care. This is especially important if the patient's home living situation is not stable or if the patient will be living alone for the first time.

If the inpatient or residential facility does not provide step-down care, options may be available in the patient's home town. At this level of care, supervision varies by facility. Facilities may provide a combination of group or individual therapy, 12-step meetings, a case worker or on-site supervisor, communal meals, curfews, and drug screenings—or none of these. Some facilities are simply a safe place to live and practice recovery. In general, there are far too few such facilities available for the vast number of patients who would benefit. A patient appropriate for this level of care will meet the standards for outpatient care, with the exception of the stable home living environment, as this will be provided by the step-down facility itself.

Ideally, an individual does not switch overnight from inpatient to outpatient care but instead is able to step down to a lower level of care over time, practicing his or her independent living skills without being totally self-reliant. This type of transitional living is common for individuals recovering from drug or alcohol dependence but rare for those recovering from eating disorders. Depending on the community resources available, many patients seek treatment away from home and then must find local providers in their home town. These patients often struggle with the enormity of the transition and the drastic decrease in daily support they receive.

A common misconception that contributes to this difficult adjustment is that patients discharged from inpatient or residential care are now "cured" and no longer practicing their eating disorder. The reality is that duration of treatment is often limited by health insurance providers, and many patients leave care before achieving a stable level of recovery or the ability to maintain it. Additionally, home life entails a higher level of stressors of all kinds, rendering the skills obtained in the sterile environment of a treatment center far less effective. It is very common for patients to regress in their recovery in the first few weeks post-discharge. It is in the best interest of the patient to have outpatient care appointments scheduled prior to discharge so that the two dietitians can communicate necessary and helpful information.

Matching a Patient to an Eating Disorder Treatment Facility

At times you may be asked to recommend a treatment facility for a particular patient. It is not possible for you to know all of the options nor which would be the best for your patient, and ultimately this must be a patient (and family) decision. You may offer guidance to your patient if you are familiar with particular facilities, but empowering your patient to research his or her options is ideal. Here are some topics you can suggest to a patient or family member who asks for your advice in choosing between treatment options. Choose the questions that are applicable to each individual's situation.

- Does the facility accept patients who are medically unstable?
- Does the facility provide medical care and medical nutritional rehabilitation when indicated?
- What is the facility's philosophy of treatment? Their nutrition philosophy? Their philosophy regarding eating disorders?
- Does the facility aid patients in finding follow-up care?
- What is the cost? What insurance coverage is available? Are payment plans available? Are charity beds available?
- What are criteria for discharge? What is the average length of stay?
- Is the facility only for patients with eating disorders or for all patients needing psychiatric care?
- Does the facility provide treatment for additional issues that patients may have, such as trauma, substance abuse, or self-harm?
- Are visitors allowed? Do visitors or family members participate in treatment?
- Does the facility have a particular religious affiliation?
- Does the facility offer a step-down program or halfway house?

A Note About Insurance Coverage for Eating Disorders

At the time of this writing, Congress is debating bills on health insurance reform. If you have filed anything more than the most basic claim, you are familiar with the time, attention, energy, and paperwork involved in obtaining reimbursement for health care. Obtaining insurance coverage for eating disorder treatment is rarely straightforward and often requires many exchanges back and forth between insurance personnel, the insured, and treaters. There are many issues.

There is no one evidence-based treatment method that guarantees successful recovery from an eating disorder. Research is, at times, difficult to translate into clinical practice and vice versa.[3-6] Therefore insurers hesitate to cover eating disorders treatment that is not proven effective.[7] The view of eating disorders as behaviors of choice persists even though the biological basis has been confirmed.[4] Mental health care coverage benefits are not always adequate for the long course of treatment that may be required. Insurers waver on whether nutrition therapy for a mental illness is "medically necessary," even though the American Psychiatric Association (APA) guidelines indicate that it is.[2]

If you work in a facility, it is likely that payment for your services is rolled into a single per diem charge. You may never know if your services are being directly reimbursed or paid for by insurance, and you may not need to know. If you work in your own practice, reimbursement is more complicated. Even if you are a provider contracted with an insurance plan, your patient's reimbursement may still depend on his or her diagnosis. For example, you may be a provider for the patient's insurance, but your services may be a covered benefit only if the patient's diagnosis is diabetes.

If you are not contracted with an insurance company, then you are an "out-of-network provider." Your patient may have different coverage for in-network and out-of-network providers. If there is no alternative provider in your area that your patient could meet with (or no other provider who is a specialist in eating disorders), their insurance company may be willing to cover your services at the in-network rate on an ad hoc basis, but only if requested by the insured (patient or family member). You and the patient's other team members may be asked to provide documentation of medical necessity for your services, including anthropometric data and a description of symptoms and recommendations. Even after all this work, there is no guarantee that the patient or family will ever receive reimbursement for your services.

Most insurance companies have two separate claim processing operations—one for medical care and one for behavioral health. As an RDN, you may find your claim bounced back and forth between the medical and behavioral sides. Often the two services are not housed in the same location, so there is no internal communication. A claim for your services filed with the medical side may be denied with a letter stating that it must be filed on the behavioral health side. This is not a guarantee that the claim will be paid by the behavioral health side. Once the claim is re-filed, a denial may come from the behavioral health office as well. Eating disorders belong under behavioral health, they will say, but RDNs belong under medical care. They will argue with you, the patient, and the family, ad infinitum.

Families have sued insurance companies for such denials and won, but change happens slowly. Mental health parity laws have been passed in many states, requiring that mental health benefits be equal to medical benefits; however, it is unclear how these laws will be enforced or if they will even cover RDN services for mental health diagnoses, such as eating disorders. The Academy of Nutrition and Dietetics, along with other organizations that focus on mental health parity for individuals with eating disorders, are working on many levels to obtain better insurance coverage for the treatment of eating disorders.

References

1. Kellogg M. When and how to refer to psychotherapy. *Weight Manage Matters*. 2008;6(2):14-15.

2. Yager J, Devlin MJ, Halmi KA, et al. *Practice Guideline for the Treatment of Patients with Eating Disorders*. 3rd ed. Arlington, VA: American Psychiatric Association; 2006.

3. Barnes S, Schwartz MB. Increasing collaboration between clinicians and researchers. *Renfrew Perspect*. 2007;(Winter):5-7.

4. Tobin DL. Research and practice in eating disorders: the clinician's dilemma. *Renfrew Perspect*. 2007;(Winter):8-10.

5. Kaye W, Grefe L. Why eating disorders research is under-funded. *Renfrew Perspect*. 2007;(Winter):3-5.

6. Banker J, Klump K. Toward a common ground: bridging the gap between research and practice in the field of eating disorders. *Renfrew Perspect*. 2007;(Winter):12-14.

7. Bunnell D. Evidence-based practice: an insurers perspective. Interview with Andrei-Claudian Jaeger, MD, Medical Director, MHN, New York and New Jersey Service Center. *Renfrew Perspect*. 2007;(Winter):10-12.

Chapter 8

Nutrition Monitoring and Evaluation

In the Nutrition Care Process (NCP), step 4 is Nutrition Monitoring and Evaluation, which is an ongoing assessment and reporting of updates in the 4 domains of nutrition assessment:

- Food/Nutrition-Related History Outcomes
- Anthropometric Measurement Outcomes
- Biochemical Data, Medical Tests, and Procedure Outcomes
- Nutrition-Focused Physical Finding Outcomes

Monitoring

The frequency with which you monitor a patient will depend on some combination of Joint Commission standards, your facility's internal protocol or policy, the level of care in which you work, your patient's wishes, your professional ethics, and simply what is possible given your workload and job expectations.

Currently there is no standard of practice for the caseload of a registered dietitian nutritionist (RDN) working with eating disorder patients. Eating disorders require a high level of acuity as well as significant nutrition intervention and frequent monitoring. It is commonly accepted in our profession that patients with eating disorders may require more of an RDN's time than patients with other diagnoses, regardless of treatment setting or level of care.

If you find that your designated work hours are not adequate for the needs of your patients with eating disorders, advocate for them and for yourself by speaking with your supervisor. You may be asked to complete a time-use study or document the time spent with each patient. Ultimately, your patients will benefit from your willingness to speak up and your desire to provide the individualized nutrition guidance that each of them needs.

Evaluation

Each time you gather additional information through any means, reflect back on your nutrition assessment, nutrition diagnoses, and recommended interventions to see if any progress or deterioration can be noted. Depending on what has or has not changed since your last evaluation, you may choose to change your nutrition diagnoses or goals.

Any time you obtain new information, make a change to the treatment plan, or meet with a patient, document your findings and recommendation in the medical record. The medical record is an essential, ongoing report; however, it is important that you do not rely on the medical record for communication. Seek out or create opportunities to communicate with the other members of the team, especially if a change (or lack of change) in nutrition status or goals is unexpected or severe, requires attention from another member of the team, or indicates a need for a different level of care.

When an individual leaves your care for any reason, facilitate the transition to the next dietitian by writing a final note, if possible. Summarize the patient's history and progress to date, including your goals and interventions and whether they have been achieved; any abnormal parameters in the four areas you are monitoring; and why the patient is leaving your care. You may also include obstacles to improvement that you have observed and any other information that will assist the dietitian in moving forward with the patient. Obtain the patient's permission (or parent or legal guardian if the patient is a minor) to release this information.

Food and Nutrient Intake

Your documentation of changes in food and nutrient intake will rely on the information provided by your patient along with any corroborating information from support persons such as family members or hospital staff who are present when your patient is eating or receiving supplemental nutrition. Based on the level of care in which you work and the abilities of each patient, you may gather information from a food diary, calorie count, medical record, photo journal, verbal recall, or other method.

In the preliminary stages of treatment, nutrition intake may take precedence, while in later stages, nutrition behaviors may be of greater importance. In a facility or hospital, where other staff document mealtime behaviors, you may limit your documentation to the basics of energy needs, nutrition intake, and nutrition-related medication side effects. In an outpatient setting or when you are the only team member familiar with eating disorders, you may also include details of compensatory behaviors, adherence to exercise recommendations or restrictions, and compliance with prescribed medication.

Always document each of these parameters relative to recommended amounts, indicating if the patient met, exceeded, or did not meet goals. Ideally your documentation stands alone each time; rather than referring back to the note written on a previous date, someone reading today's note should be able to have all the information to determine if each parameter is improving or deteriorating.

If an individual was unable to meet nutrition goals, specify if you recommend continuation of current interventions or if you recommend taking a different approach moving forward. Your revised recommendations may include different delivery methods, additional support at mealtimes, a change in texture or diet type, and any other parameters that will assist your patient in reaching any goals that were not met in the previous time period.

You may determine that certain nutritional goals are no longer needed, either because they have been met, the underlying issue has been resolved, or your patient's needs have changed. Use information in the medical record and from your communication with other members of the treatment team to determine if a nutrition diagnosis is no longer applicable or if a change in the patient's health status requires that a new nutrition diagnosis (and associated interventions) take precedence.

It would be ideal if every time you follow up with a patient, you learn that your recommendations are being followed, and your patient's nutrition status is improving. Unfortunately the mental illness aspect of eating disorders makes perfect adherence to your meal plan unlikely unless your patient is supervised at all times. An eating disorder impairs a patient's ability to assess his or her own compliance as well as awareness of crucial features of the meal plan, such as portion size, food preparation method, and whether the meal was completed or not.

Discrepancies between what you recommend and what your patient actually eats are caused by the eating disorder disease process, but as a new RDN, it can be difficult not to take them personally. It's important to remember your patient may be experiencing paralyzing feelings of anxiety, ambivalence, or dread surrounding what to others is just eating. Keep in mind that if eating appropriately was easy for this patient, he or she would never have arrived in your care. This may help you retain compassion for your patient during periods when food and nutrient intake does not improve. When you observe a continued lack of improvement, discuss with the treatment team the possible need for a higher level of care.

Anthropometrics

In theory, anthropometric data would be the easiest way to observe and document an individual's progress or lack of progress during eating disorder treatment. In reality it can also be the most inconclusive or even deceptive piece to monitor and evaluate, especially since body weight is (rightly or wrongly) both the most commonly used anthropometric measurement and the easiest to misinterpret.

The anxiety associated with eating disorders can prompt a patient who is undereating to manipulate his or her body weight in order to meet designated weight goals or please the treatment team or family members or to allow the patient to continue to lose weight without detection. Drinking fluids prior to being weighed, known as water-loading, is only one of many means an individual can use to deceive the scale. Concealing foreign objects in pockets or within undergarments or wearing multiple layers of clothes can at least be circumvented, for the most part, by weighing each patient in a hospital-type gown. Over time, and especially if weights fluctuate in short periods outside normal body weight expectations, unnatural methods of manipulating weight usually are revealed. However, rapid weight changes should not be discounted, as they can also be symptoms of renal failure, cardiac failure, edema, protein-malnutrition, and other serious conditions.

If your facility has more than one scale or a patient is being weighed in more than one medical office, arrange for only one scale to be used, otherwise inaccuracy between scales will impair your ability to evaluate what is a weight change versus what is a calibration error.

Adding to the difficulty of evaluating anthropometrics is the lens of eating disorders that can cause the same information to be interpreted quite differently by the treatment team and by the patient. For example, a physician may express relief that a patient's weight is "out of the danger zone," while the patient understands this to signify that he or she is no longer thin enough. Patients have also reported equating the word healthy with fat, and well-meaning comments such as "You are looking much better," as "You have gained weight."

In light of this ability to misinterpret what you may previously have thought of as harmless or even complimentary comments, it is wise in many cases to simply document biometric information, particularly body weight, within the medical record rather than discussing it with the patient. Focus your nutrition counseling on the actions and behaviors that you are recommending for a patient rather than a weight goal that you would like the patient to achieve.

The same approach is equally appropriate for patients who are striving to lose weight. In cases where an individual equates body weight with self-worth and value, a failure to lose weight over a certain period of time can be perceived as proof that nutrition interventions are ineffective.

In some cases, you may find yourself educating not only your patients but also family members and other health professionals about the normal fluctuations of weight and reassuring them that consistency in eating behaviors is the only way toward lasting change. Assisting a patient who is weighing him or herself daily or more frequently to decrease reliance on the scale for reassurance is a task that you and the mental health professional on the team can undertake together.

Ultimately the key component of documenting anthropometric changes is to put them into context. For example, in addition to noting a patient's current weight and weight change since your last evaluation, include how the patient's current weight compares with your recommendation, your explanation of why the weight change occurred, whether the change is a beneficial or detrimental, and of course whether your nutrition recommendations are the same or different based on this information.

Biochemical Data, Medical Tests, and Procedures

The results of some medical tests and procedures may influence your nutrition diagnoses and interventions if they are nutrition-related or have a nutritional impact. It is important to know the period over which changes can be expected so that you can monitor them at appropriate intervals. For example, a low blood glucose level is a useful indicator of malnutrition in the short term and may normalize almost immediately upon eating, while a low albumin level is a longer-term indicator of malnutrition and takes approximately 6 weeks to improve. If you are not familiar with a given procedure or test, or what it signifies, find out if there is any nutritional impact by asking a member of the treatment team or another dietitian, or with your own research.

Monitoring and evaluating laboratory values are also important but potentially deceptive. You are now aware that in many cases of eating disorders, laboratory values remain within normal limits even when a patient is very malnourished and ill. It is difficult to document improvement in laboratory values if they were never out of range to begin with. You may find that medical providers unfamiliar with eating disorders, as well as patients and family members, look to normal or low normal laboratory values as confirmation that a patient is no longer or never was ill, or that the patient's eating disorder is not severe enough to need treatment.

When a malnourished person begins the refeeding process, frequent, even daily monitoring of certain laboratory values becomes essential. It is only once the acute deficiencies begin to resolve that the chronic deficiencies are revealed, and dangerously low levels of electrolytes can result. Although these laboratory tests are measuring nutrient deficiencies, the deficiencies are so severe that they cannot be corrected with food. Therefore the medical provider on your team will be responsible for monitoring these laboratory values and prescribing the therapeutic oral or intravenous supplementation that will be required.

Nutrition-Focused Physical Findings

Many of the nutrition-focused physical findings associated with eating disorders are slow to improve and will not have changed from one follow-up visit to another. The exceptions are vital signs, such as heart rate and blood pressure, which can change depending on hydration status, body position, and physical activity. If an individual is in jeopardy, ideally he or she will be monitored closely and restricted from exercise; however, in reality, individuals with eating disorders may be ambulatory even when severely compromised. If you observe a patient looking flushed or faint while seated or when rising from seated to standing, communicate immediately with the medical provider on the team for guidance.

The benefit to the slow pace of change of the majority of the other physical findings is that when they resolve, it is a clear sign of improvement. For example, when patients report that their hair is no longer falling out, that food is tasting better, that the daily headache is only once in a while, that they are no longer experiencing constipation, when you can no longer see a patient's temple bones, or when a patient's lips are pink instead of blue—these are all indications that your nutritional interventions are having their desired effect over the long term and worthy of noting in the medical record.

Not all improvements are so happily welcomed by patients. In some cases they may think that getting healthier means that they are no longer successful at their eating disorder. This should be reported to the mental health professional on the team. It will be a challenge that patients will need all available support to overcome.

Ultimately each individual will heal and recover at a different pace, sometimes happily and productively and sometimes discouragingly slowly. Sadly there are also patients who will not be able to recover at all, but as treatment modalities and our understanding of eating disorders improves, hopefully this number will decrease.

As you progress in your work with individuals with eating disorders, you will undoubtedly have many satisfying experiences, and, more than likely, you will have some discouraging ones as well. In the best case scenario, you will eventually be able to document that your initial nutrition diagnoses have been resolved and your patients' nutrition goals have been achieved.

Appendix A

Nutrition Care Process Summary

THE NUTRITION CARE PROCESS MODEL

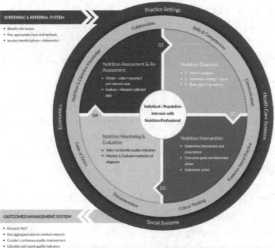

Reprinted with permission from the Academy of Nutrition and Dietetics. Nutrition assessment introduction. In: *Nutrition Terminology Reference Manual (eNCPT): Dietetics Language for Nutrition Care*. Nutrition Care Process Introduction. http://ncpt.webauthor.com/pubs/idnt-en/

Four Steps in Nutrition Care Process

Step 1: Nutrition Assessment

Obtain, verify, and interpret data needed to identify nutrition-related problems, their causes, and significance.

Step 2: Nutrition Diagnosis

Identify and describe a specific nutrition problem that can be resolved or improved through treatment/nutrition intervention by a food and nutrition professional. The nutrition diagnosis is conveyed in a problem, etiology, symptoms (PES) statement.

Step 3: Nutrition Intervention

Resolve or improve the nutrition diagnosis or nutrition problem by provision of advice, education, or delivery of the food component of a specific diet or meal plan tailored to the patient's need. The interventions are directed at the etiology of the diagnosis (PES statement).

Step 4: Nutrition Monitoring and Evaluation

Determine and measure the amount of progress made for the nutrition intervention and whether the nutrition-related goals/outcomes are being met, thus, determining the effectiveness of the interventions by selecting care indicators and the criteria to which the indicator is compared.

Adapted from the Academy of Nutrition and Dietetics. Nutrition assessment introduction. In: *Nutrition Terminology Reference Manual (eNCPT): Dietetics Language for Nutrition Care.* Nutrition Care Process Introduction. http://ncpt.webauthor.com/pubs/idnt-en/

Appendix B

Guide to Restrictive Eating Styles

As with any patient population, patients with eating disorders may adhere to a restricted eating style, such as vegetarian, halal, or gluten free. Rationale for these eating restrictions varies and may include desired weight loss, religious tradition, medical necessity, family practices, disease prevention, personal moral and ethical beliefs, environmental concerns, and personal choice. There may also be more socially acceptable terminology for the eating disorder. It may take time to pick apart the distinction.

Depending on how and why each patient applies restrictions, you may determine that the restrictions are not nutritionally adequate or appropriate to promote recovery. Each facility should have a standard policy in place for handling patient food preferences at admission. If a facility does not allow vegetarian eating, for example, or does not have a kosher kitchen, this should be clearly stated so that patient and family can make an informed choice of whether their needs can be met.

Table B.1 provides the standard guidelines for a variety of restrictive eating styles. In some cases, a patient may not actually or strictly follow the restrictive eating style he or she subscribes to. It is, therefore, important to investigate each patient's actual food preferences so that the meal plan is not unnecessarily restricted. In addition, a patient may be willing to relax his or her eating standards temporarily if this will improve the patient's chances or rate of recovery.

Personal preferences should always be treated with respect; however, if it is in the patient's best interest to include some formerly excluded foods, this topic can be appropriately broached by the registered dietitian nutrition-ist. Most eating styles, including those founded on religious beliefs, allow latitude in light of medical needs. For example, a member of the Muslim faith is allowed to eat nonhalal food if no halal food is available; a member of the Jewish faith is not allowed to fast on even the most holy of fast days if it will harm his or her health. Patients who are struggling with religious beliefs that conflict with their need for eating disorder treatment may benefit from referral to a religious leader of their faith who can help reconcile the conflict or grant permission to follow medical advice that seems to contradict with religious teachings.

Table B.1 Restrictive Eating Styles

Name	Excludes	Includes	Rationale
Semivegetarian	All beef, pork, and their products	Poultry Eggs Seafood Dairy	Varies by individual; motivation may be health-related, animal rights-based, or linked to a past bad experience with a restricted food
Pesco-vegetarian	Beef, pork, poultry, and their products	Seafood Dairy Eggs	
Lacto-ovo vegetarian	Beef, pork, poultry, and their products Seafood	Dairy Eggs	
Lacto-vegetarian	Beef, pork, poultry, and their products Seafood Eggs	Dairy	
Vegan	All animal products	All plant foods	

Continued on next page.

Table B.1 (cont.) Restrictive Eating Styles

Name	Excludes	Includes	Rationale
Macrobiotic	All animal products Certain fruits and juice Coffee Processed foods Artificial ingredients	Beans Vegetables Tofu Whole grains Tea	Live "in balance with nature" for a healthy mind, body, and spirit
Calorie restricting	Processed sugars Flour "Calorie-sparse" foods Red meat White rice	Vegetables Small amounts of fish Nutrition supplements	Eat as few calories as possible of nutrient-dense foods in an effort to prolong lifespan
Raw foods	Cooked food Processed food Food heated to > 116°F	Vegetables Fruits (fresh or dried) Sprouts Nuts and seeds Grains Beans Seaweed	Heating food destroys digestive enzymes in food; cooking diminishes the nutritional value and life-force of food

Continued on next page.

Table B.1 (cont.) Restrictive Eating Styles

Name	Excludes	Includes	Rationale
Kashrus/Kahsrut, also called keeping kosher or kosher	Pork and all pork products (includes pork gelatin) Shellfish Dairy and meat of any kind in the same meal Beef and poultry not certified kosher	All fruits and vegetables Dairy products Fish Beef and poultry certified kosher Packaged food with kosher symbols	Jewish religious belief prescribed in the Hebrew Bible. Note: Kashrus is not followed by everyone of the Jewish faith—assess on an individual basis before ordering a kosher diet
Halal	Pork and all pork products (includes pork gelatin) Alcohol in any form	All fruits and vegetables Dairy products Fish Beef and poultry certified halal or kosher	Muslim religious belief prescribed in the Koran. Note: Halal is not followed by every-one of the Muslim faith—assess on an individual basis
Lent (Christian Orthodox)	No animal foods are allowed from Ash Wednesday through Easter, except on Sundays	Vegetarian diet daily Unrestricted diet on Sundays	Christian religious belief practiced by members of certain Christian Orthodox faiths

Continued on next page.

Table B.1 (cont.) Restrictive Eating Styles

Name	Excludes	Includes	Rationale
Lent (Roman Catholic)	Meat from hooved animals (beef and pork) not allowed on Fridays from Ash Wednesday through Easter	Unrestricted diet daily Fish and dairy allowed on Fridays	Christian religious belief practiced by members of the Roman Catholic faith. Note: practices vary widely—assess on an individual basis
Lent (Protestant)	Each individual chooses something to "give up for Lent," the period from Ash Wednesday through Easter	Food not required to be restricted; another activity, such as gossip, or another bad habit may be chosen	Christian religious belief practiced by members of certain Protestant faiths. Note: practices vary widely—assess on an individual basis
Paleo	Cereal grains, legumes (including peanuts) Dairy Refined sugar Potatoes Processed foods Salt Refined vegetable oils	Grass-fed meats Fish and seafood Fresh fruits Vegetables Eggs Nuts and seeds Olive, walnut, flaxseed, macadamia, avocado, and coconut oils	Based on the premise that an optimal diet is what our distant ancestors ate before the advent of agriculture (during the Paleolithic period, hence the name)

Continued on next page.

Table B.1 (cont.) Restrictive Eating Styles

Name	Excludes	Includes	Rationale
Gluten free	Wheat, rye, barley, and all foods containing them, their flour, or their gluten storage proteins: gliadin, secalin and hordein Most baked goods, pastas, and cereals Processed foods with gluten-related ingredients	All meats Fish Poultry Eggs Corn, quinoa, rice Legumes Nuts and seeds Dairy Fruits Vegetables Baked goods and pasta made from gluten-free flours Malt vinegar	Medical diet for celiac disease, also called gluten-intolerance Has been adopted by celebrities and touted as a fad diet for weight loss and general health. Following a gluten-free diet prior to diagnosis with celiac disease can confound test results and cause a false-negative reading

Appendix C

Caffeine Content in Common Foods, Beverages, and Drugs

Coffees	Serving Size	Caffeine (mg)
Dunkin' Donuts Coffee with Turbo Shot	20 fl oz	436
Dunkin' Donuts Cappuccino	20 fl oz	151
Dunkin' Donuts Coffee	14 fl oz	178
Dunkin' Donuts, Panera, or Starbucks Decaf Coffee	16 fl oz	15–25
Folgers Classic Roast Instant Coffee	2 tsp	148
International Delight Iced Cof-fee	8 fl oz	76
Keurig Coffee K-Cup, all varieties	1 pod	75–150
Maxwell House Decaf Ground Coffee	2 Tbs	2–10
Maxwell House Ground Coffee 100% Colombian, Dark Roast, Master Blend, or Original Roast	2 Tbs	100–160
Maxwell House International Café, all flavors	2 Tbs	40–130
Maxwell House Lite Ground Coffee	2 Tbs	50–70
McDonald's Coffee	16 fl oz	133
Panera Coffee	16.8 fl oz	189
Panera Frozen Mocha	16.5 fl oz	267
Seattle's Best Coffee—Iced Latte or Iced Mocha, can	9.5 fl oz	90
Starbucks Caffè Americano	6 fl oz	225

Continued on next page.

Coffees (cont.)	Serving Size	Caffeine (mg)
Starbucks Caffè Mocha	6 fl oz	175
Starbucks Coffee	16 fl oz	330
	20 fl oz	415
Starbucks Coffee	12 fl oz	260
Starbucks Doubleshot Energy Coffee, can	15 fl oz	146
Starbucks Espresso	doppio (2 fl oz)	150
Starbucks Espresso Frappuccino	24 fl oz	185
Starbucks Frappuccino Coffee, bottle	9.5 fl oz	90
Starbucks Iced Coffee	6 fl oz	165
Starbucks Mocha Frappuccino	24 fl oz	140
Starbucks VIA House Blend Instant Coffee	1 packet	135
Starbucks—Caffè Latte, Cappuccino, or Caramel Macchiato	16 fl oz	150

Teas	Serving Size	Caffeine (mg)
Arizona Iced Tea, black, all varieties	16 fl oz	30
Arizona Iced Tea, green, all varieties	16 fl oz	15
Black tea, brewed for 3 minutes	8 fl oz	30–80
Green tea, brewed for 3 minutes	8 fl oz	35–60
Herbal tea, brewed	8 fl oz	0
Lipton 100% Natural Lemon Iced Tea, bottle	20 fl oz	35

Continued on next page.

Teas (cont.)	Serving Size	Caffeine (mg)
Lipton Decaffeinated Tea—black or green, brewed	8 fl oz	5
Lipton Pure Leaf Iced Tea	18.5 fl oz	60
Nestea Unsweetened Iced Tea Mix	2 tsp	20–30
Snapple Lemon Tea	16 fl oz	62
Starbucks Tazo Awake—Brewed Tea or Tea Latte	16 fl oz	135
Starbucks Tazo Chai Tea Latte	16 fl oz	95
Starbucks Tazo Earl Grey—Brewed Tea or Tea Latte	16 fl oz	115
Starbucks Tazo Green Tea Latte—Iced or regular	6 fl oz	80

Soft Drinks[a]	Serving Size	Caffeine (mg)
7-Up, Fanta, Fresca, ginger ale, or Sprite	12 oz.	0
Barq's Root Beer, regular	12 oz 20 oz	23
Coca-Cola Life	12 oz 20 oz	27 45
Coca-Cola, Coke Zero, or Diet Pepsi	12 oz 20 oz	35 58
Diet Coke	12 oz 20 oz	47 78
Dr Pepper or Sunkist, regular or diet	12 oz 20 oz	41 68
Mountain Dew, regular or diet	12 oz 20 oz	54 90
Mountain Zevia (Zevia)	12 oz	55

Continued on next page.

Soft Drinks (cont.)	Serving Size	Caffeine (mg)
Pepsi	12 oz	38
	20 oz	63
Pepsi MAX	12 oz	69
Pepsi True	7.5 oz	24
	20 oz	64
Root beer, most brands, or Barq's Diet Root Beer	12 oz 20 oz	0
Surge	8 oz	35
	20 oz	87

Energy Drinks	Serving Size	Caffeine (mg)
5-hour Energy	1.9 fl oz	208
AMP Energy Boost Original (PepsiCo)	16 fl oz	142
Ávitãe Caffeinated Water	16.9 fl oz	90
Bang Energy Drink	16 fl oz	357
Frava Caffeinated Juice	16 oz	200
Full Throttle (Monster)	16 fl oz	200
Glacéau Vitaminwater Energy	20 fl oz	50
Monster Energy	16 fl oz	160
Mountain Dew Kick Start	16 fl oz	92
NoDoz Energy Shots	1.89 fl oz	115
NOS Energy Drink (Monster)	16 fl oz	160
Ocean Spray Cran-Energy	20 fl oz	55
Red Bull	8.4 fl oz	80
Redline Energy Drink	8 fl oz	316
Rockstar	16 fl oz	160
Rockstar Citrus Punched	16 fl oz	240
Starbucks Refreshers	12 fl oz	50

Continued on next page.

Energy Drinks (cont.)	Serving Size	Caffeine (mg)
V8 V-Fusion+Energy	8 fl oz	80
Venom Energy Drink (Dr Pepper/Seven Up Inc.)	16 fl oz	160

Frozen Desserts	Serving Size	Caffeine (mg)
Bang!! Caffeinated Ice Cream	4 fl oz	125
Baskin Robbins Jamoca Ice Cream	4 fl oz	20
Breyers Coffee Ice Cream	4 fl oz	1
Cold Stone Creamery Mocha Ice Cream	12 fl oz	52
Dannon All Natural Coffee Lowfat Yogurt	6 oz	30
Dreyer's or Edy's Grand Ice Cream—Coffee or Espresso Chip	4 fl oz	17
Dreyer's, Edy's, or Häagen-Dazs Chocolate Ice Cream	4 fl oz	less than 1
Häagen-Dazs Coffee Almond Crunch Snack Size Bar	1.8 oz	10
Häagen-Dazs Coffee Ice Cream	4 fl oz	29
Starbucks Coffee Ice Cream	4 fl oz	45
Starbucks Mocha Frappuccino Ice Cream	4 fl oz	25
Stonyfield Gotta Have Java Nonfat Frozen Yogurt	4 fl oz	28
TCBY Coffee Frozen Yogurt	13.4 fl oz	42

Continued on next page.

Chocolates/Candies/Other	Serving Size	Caffeine (mg))
Awake Caffeinated Chocolate Bar	1.55 oz	101
Awake Caffeinated Chocolate Bites	0.53 oz	50
Blue Diamond Almonds, Roasted Coffee Flavored	1 oz	25
Crackheads	1 box, 40g	600
Crackheads Espresso Bean Candies, regular	1 package (28 pieces)	200
Crystal Light Energy	½ packet	60
Dove Dark Chocolate Silky Smooth Promises	5 pieces,	4
Hershey's Cocoa	1 Tbs	8
Hershey's Kisses	9 pieces	9
Hershey's Special Dark Chocolate Bar	1.5 oz	20
Hershey's—Milk Chocolate Bar	1.6 oz	9
Jelly Belly Extreme Sport Beans	1 package	50
Jolt Gum	1 piece	45
MiO Energy, all flavors	1 squirt, ½ tsp.	60
Muscle Milk Orange Energy Chews	1.27 oz	30
Perky Jerky	1 oz	10
Silk Chocolate Soymilk	8 fl oz	4
Starbucks Hot Chocolate	16 fl oz	25
Wired Waffles	1 waffle	200

Continued on next page.

Over-The-Counter Drugs	Serving Size	Caffeine (mg)
Anacin	2 tablets	64
Bayer Back & Body	2 caplets	65
Excedrin Migraine	2 tablets	130
Midol Complete	2 caplets	120
NoDoz or Vivarin	1 caplet	200
Zantrex-3 weight-loss supplement	2 capsules	300

[a] The US Food and Drug Administration sets the limit for cola and pepper soft drinks at 71 mg (200 parts per million) per 12oz serving.

Adapted with permission from the Center for Science in the Public Interest. Caffeine chart. https://cspinet.org/eating-healthy/ingredients-of-concern/caffeine-chart. Accessed August 22, 2016.

Additional information: Juliano LM, Griffiths RR. Caffeine. In: Lowinson JH, Ruiz P, Millman RB, Langrod JG, eds. *Substance Abuse: A Comprehensive Textbook.* 4th ed. Baltimore: Lippincott, Williams & Wilkins; 2005:403-421.

Appendix D

Additional Resources

Books, Workshops, and Resources from Dietitians

A New View of Eating Disorders: Dietitians and Family-Based Treatment, by Melanie Jacob, www.melanie jacob.com

Comprehensive Learning Teaching Handout Series on CD, by Sondra Kronberg, www.sondrakronberg.com

Eating Disorder Nutrition Therapy Training, by Marci Anderson Evans, www.marcird.com

Eating Disorders Boot Camp Home-Study Course, Training Workshop for Professionals; Advanced Eating Disorders Boot Camp: Special Forces Training Home-Study Course; and Eating Disorders Nutrition Counseling DVD, by Jessica Setnick, www .understandingnutrition.com

Food–Medication Interactions Handbook, 17th edition, by Zaneta Pronsky and Sr Jeanne Patricia Crowe, www .foodmedinteractions.com

Forms, handouts, and worksheets for work with eating disorders, by Lori Pereyra, www.nutritiousways.com

Francie White Inner Escapes workshops, www.dranita johnston.com/workshops

Intuitive Eating: A Revolutionary Program That Works, revised edition; and professional trainings, by Evelyn Tribole and Elyse Resch, www.intuitiveeating.com

Love Your Body: Change the Way You Feel About the Body You Have, by Tami Brannon-Quan and Lisa Licavoli.

Molly Kellogg's Counseling Intensive for Nutrition Professionals workshop; *Counseling Tips for Nutrition Therapists: Practice Workbook Series*, Volumes 1 and 2, by Molly Kellogg, www.mollykellogg.com

Moving Away from Diets: Healing Eating Problems and Exercise Resistance, 2nd edition, by Karin Kratina, Nancy King, and Dayle Hayes, www.helmpublishing.com

Nancy Clark's Sports Nutrition Guidebook, 5th edition, by Nancy Clark, www.nancyclarkrd.com

Nutrition Counseling and Communication Skills, by Katharine Curry and Amy Jaffe

Nutrition Counseling in the Treatment of Eating Disorders, 2nd edition, by Marcia Herrin and Maria Larkin,

PCOS: The Dietitian's Guide, 2nd edition, by Angela Grassi

The PCOS Workbook: Your Guide to Complete Physical and Emotional Health, by Angela Grassi and Stephanie Mattei

The PCOS Nutrition Center Cookbook: 100 Easy and Delicious Whole Food Recipes to Beat PCOS, by Angela Grassi and Natalie Zaparzynski, www.PCOSnutrition.com

Pediatric Nutrition in Chronic Diseases and Developmental Disorders: Prevention, Assessment, and Treatment, 2nd edition, and coordinating self-study program, by Shirley W. Ekvall and Valli K. Ekvall

Winning the War Within: Nutrition Therapy for Clients with Eating Disorders, 2nd edition, by Eileen Stellefson Myers

Eating Disorder Professional, Educational and Advocacy Organizations

The Academy for Eating Disorders (AED), http://www.aedweb.org/

Adios Barbie, http://www.adiosbarbie.com/

Anorexia Nervosa and Associated Disorders (ANAD),
  http://www.anad.org/

ASPIRE, http://aspire-network.blogspot.com/2014/02
  /welcome-to-aspire.html

Association Anorexia Nervosa Bulimia Nervosa (ANBN)
  Belgium, www.anbn.be

Anorexia and Bulimia Quebec (ANEB), http://www
  .anebquebec.com/html/en/home/home.html

Australian and New Zealand Academy for Eating Disorders (ANZAED), http://www.anzaed.org.au/

Beating Eating Disorders, www.facebook.com
  /spreadingawarenesswhereitsneeded

BingeBehavior.com, http://bingebehavior.com/

Binge Eating Disorder Association (BEDA), http://beda
  online.com/

Bullemia.com, www.bulimia.com

The Butterfly Foundation, http://www.thebutterfly
  foundation.org.au/

The Dirty Laundry Project (DLP), https://www.facebook.
  com/Dirtylaundryproject

Eating Disorders Coalition, www.eatingdisorders
  coalition.org

Eating Disorder Hope (resources for coping with eating
  disorders), www.eatingdisorderhope.com

Eating Disorder Jobs (resources for professionals and job
  seekers), www.eatingdisorderjobs.com

Eating Disorder Parent Support (EDPS), http://eating
  disorderparentsupport.weebly.com/

Eating Disorders Association of New Zealand, (EDANZ),
  www.ed.org.nz

Eating Disorders Victoria (EDV), http://www.eating
  disorders.org.au

Elephant in the Room Foundation, https://www.EitRF.org/

International Association of Eating Disorders Professionals Foundation, www.iaedp.com

International Eating Disorders Action (IEDAction),
http://iedaction.weebly.com/

International Federation of Eating Disorder Dietitians,
www.ifedd.com

Islam and Eating Disorders, Maya Khan, http://waragainst
eatingdisorder.com/

Michelle's Voice: The Society for Eating Disorder Awareness and Education, https://twitter.com/dmichellestory

Men Get Eating Disorders Too (MGEDT), http://menget
edstoo.co.uk/

Mentor Connect: Relationships Replace Eating Disorders,
www.mentorconnect-ed.org

Multi-Service Eating Disorder Association, (MEDA),
http://www.medainc.org/

National Association for Males with Eating Disorders
(NAMED), http://namedinc.org/

National Eating Disorder Association (NEDA), http://
www.nationaleatingdisorders.org/

National Eating Disorder Collaboration, Australia www
.nedc.com.au/

National Eating Disorder Information Centre (NEDIC),
http://nedic.ca/

National Initiative for Eating Disorders, (NIED), http://
nied.ca/

Project Heal, http://theprojectheal.org/chapters-heal
/toronto/

ReGlam Me, http://www.reglam.me/, Germany and global

SockIt to ED campaign, https://www.facebook.com
/events/1517755561812119/

The Renfrew Center Foundation, http://renfrewcenter
.com/renfrew-center-foundation

Trans Folx Fighting Eating Disorders (T-FFED),
www.transfolxfightingeds.org/

Eating Disorder Certification Programs for Dietitians

Certified Eating Disorders Registered Dietitian (CEDRD), www.iaedp.com

CEDRD Certification Prep Class, by Jessica Setnick, www.CEDRD.com

Postgraduate Intensive Training for Dietitians Treating Eating Disorders, by the Institute for Contemporary Psychotherapy Center for the Study of Anorexia and Bulimia (ICP CSAB), http://icpnyc.org/csab/2-year -training-program

Index

Page number followed by *b* signifies box; *t*, table.